Clinical 3 T Magnetic Resonance

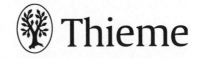

Clinical 3 T Magnetic Resonance

Val M. Runge, M.D.
Robert and Alma Moreton Centennial Chair in Radiology
Department of Radiology
Scott & White Clinic and Hospital
Texas A&M Health Science Center
Temple, Texas

Wolfgang R. Nitz, Ph.D.
Application Development
MR Division
Siemens Medical Solutions
Erlangen, Germany

Stuart H. Schmeets, B.S., R.T.(R)(MR)
Advanced Specialist Ultra High-Field MRI Applications
Siemens Medical Solutions USA, Inc.
Malvern, Pennsylvania

Stefan O. Schoenberg, M.D.
Associate Professor of Radiology
Associate Chair of Clinical Operations
Department of Clinical Radiology
University Hospitals-Grosshadern
Ludwig-Maximilians-University Munich
Munich, Germany

Thieme
New York • Stuttgart

Thieme Medical Publishers, Inc.
333 Seventh Ave.
New York, NY 10001

Editorial Assistant: David Price
Executive Editor: Timothy Hiscock
Vice President, Production and Electronic Publishing: Anne T. Vinnicombe
Production Editor: Shannon Kerner
Associate Marketing Manager: Verena Diem
Sales Director: Ross Lumpkin
Chief Financial Officer: Peter van Woerden
President: Brian D. Scanlan
Compositor: Thomson Press Ltd.
Printer: Maple–Vail Book Manufacturing Group

Library of Congress Cataloging-in-Publication Data

Runge, Val M.
  Clinical 3 T magnetic resonance / Val M. Runge . . . [et al.].
    p. ; cm.
  Includes index.
  ISBN 1–58890–403–2 (pbk. : alk. paper) — ISBN 3–13–141101–5 (pbk. : alk. paper)
  1. Magnetic resonance imaging. I. Runge, Val M. II. Title: Clinical three tesla magnetic resonance.
  [DNLM: 1. Magnetic Resonance Imaging—methods. WN 185 C6418 2006]
  RC78.7.N83.C555 2006
  616.07'548—dc22

                                              2006022259

Important note: Medical knowledge is ever-changing. As new research and clinical experience broaden our knowledge, changes in treatment and drug therapy may be required. The authors and editors of the material herein have consulted sources believed to be reliable in their efforts to provide information that is complete and in accord with the standards accepted at the time of publication. However, in view of the possibility of human error by the authors, editors, or publisher of the work herein or changes in medical knowledge, neither the authors, editors, nor publisher, nor any other party who has been involved in the preparation of this work, warrants that the information contained herein is in every respect accurate or complete, and they are not responsible for any errors or omissions or for the results obtained from use of such information. Readers are encouraged to confirm the information contained herein with other sources. For example, readers are advised to check the product information sheet included in the package of each drug they plan to administer to be certain that the information contained in this publication is accurate and that changes have not been made in the recommended dose or in the contraindications for administration. This recommendation is of particular importance in connection with new or infrequently used drugs.

Some of the product names, patents, and registered designs referred to in this book are in fact registered trademarks or proprietary names even though specific reference to this fact is not always made in the text. Therefore, the appearance of a name without designation as proprietary is not to be construed as a representation by the publisher that it is in the public domain.

Printed in the United States of America

5 4 3 2 1

TMP ISBN 1-58890-403-2
TMP ISBN 978-1-58890-403-4
GTV ISBN 3 13 141101 5
GTV ISBN 978-3-13-141101-3

To my father, who passed away during the writing of this book, and to his loving wife of 59 years, my mother, who both were the inspiration for my career, and to my two daughters, Sadie and Valerie, with all my love.

With special thanks to John E. Kirsch, Ph.D., for his detailed explanations of subject material throughout the course of development of this book.

I would also like to express my sincere appreciation to the many members of the Radiology Department at Scott & White, and in particular Jilene Gendron, who by their hard work and support made this project possible.

Contents

Foreword

Clinical magnetic resonance imaging (MRI) is clearly moving from 1.5 T to 3 T. With the higher field comes better signal-to-noise ratios (SNR) that can be used for higher spatial resolution, thinner slices, or faster scanning. Given the 10-year lifespan of most MRI systems, anyone not purchasing a 3 T instead of a 1.5 T MRI system today either doesn't have the patient volume or the dollars to justify it financially, or is afraid of the physics.

Val M. Runge, M.D., and his colleagues have put together an excellent book discussing the implications (from a physics standpoint) of going from 1.5 T to 3 T and making their points with numerous comparisons of the same lesions taken from all areas of the body examined at both fields.

The physics discussion presented in this book is both understandable and relevant. The authors discuss the advantages of going to 3 T, one of which is its synergy with parallel imaging which allows the user to trade-off the extra SNR at 3 T for faster scanning or reduced susceptibility effects. To be more specific, the extra SNR at 3 T allows for scanning four times as fast, all other parameters staying the same. Diamagnetic susceptibility effects at 3 T, for example, the distortion over the petrous bones on EPI diffusion images, can be reduced to 1.5 T levels through use of parallel imaging.

The authors also discuss the disadvantages of 3 T and tricks to get around them. Without modification, the radio-frequency (RF) heating increases the specific absorption rate (SAR) by a factor of 4. But by reducing the flip angle of the 180 degrees refocusing pulses of a fast-spin echo exam to approximately 120 degrees, the RF heating is reduced. Dielectric effects are also discussed. These effects, which are minimal at 1.5 T, can lead to artifacts at 3 T. When the wavelength of the radiowave approaches the dimensions of the body, leading to standing waves, these result in areas of high or low signal intensity.

In summary, Dr. Runge and his coauthors have done an excellent job describing the differences between the premium platform of the last 20 years (1.5 T) and that of the next 20 years (3 T). They show that 3 T MRI is clearly ready for prime time. After reading this book, you will agree.

William G. Bradley Jr., M.D., Ph.D., F.A.C.R.
Professor and Chairman
Department of Radiology
University of California, San Diego
San Diego, California

Foreword

When considering the field of 3 T MR, one has to ask: "What can I buy at 3 T?" Certainly, increased signal-to-noise ratio (SNR) is a major benefit. Many may debate whether a factor-of-two improvement is actually achieved. Regardless, increased SNR is a given. Due to the increase in SNR, certain types of scans can be acquired at 3 T that are simply not feasible at 1.5 T. High in-plane spatial resolution diffusion-weighted imaging is one of many examples. The improvement in SNR affords the ability to substantially decrease scan time and to increase spatial resolution. Tissue properties are altered as well with the increase in main magnetic field. T1 relaxation times lengthen, and magnetic susceptibility effects increase. Although some may view these changes as problems, they can be advantageous when scanning parameters are optimized for 3 T.

Patient safety is certainly an issue that must be considered when imaging patients at 3 T. Implants and devices that have been tested and found safe at lower fields need to be tested at 3 T. The force exerted on a ferromagnetic object is greatly influenced by magnet design in addition to field strength. A cautionary note is that the fringe magnetic field on modern 3 T systems is deceptively small and relatively close to the unit due to shielding. Lastly, new implants and devices are introduced continually. Safety policies need to be reviewed and updated often. So-called blanket policies are not wise for any field strength. As with any MR system, controlling access to the MR suite is paramount.

Other safety considerations, to a certain degree, are no different than those seen at lower fields. Gradient switching rates, for example, are essentially the same as most high-end 1.5 T systems. Gradient acoustic noise increases with B_0. However, improved gradient coil designs keep this increase to a minimum. While we do not exceed the current specific absorption rate (SAR) limits, we do reach that limit more rapidly at 3 T because SAR increases with the square of the magnetic field.

The SAR issue can certainly be challenging at 3 T. It is not, however, insurmountable. Of greatest importance has been the development of imaging approaches that lower SAR. Examples, as detailed in the chapters of this book, include SPACE and VERSE. The former involves a modification of the flip angles used for signal refocusing, and the latter employs a time-varying gradient waveform. Substantial reductions in SAR can be achieved while maintaining tissue contrast with little if any loss in SNR.

The prolongation of T1 seen at 3 T provides improved image contrast in several clinical situations. The increased saturation of background tissue in three-dimensional time-of-flight MR angiography sequences results in improved contrast between flow and background.

Cardiac tagging sequences benefit as the saturation bands "linger" longer over the cardiac cycle. Perfusion techniques using arterial spin-labeling are more effective.

The increase in magnetic susceptibility effect at 3 T as compared with 1.5 T results in increased sensitivity to hemorrhage and its residual products, specifically deoxyhemoglobin, intracellular methemoglobin, and hemosiderin. The BOLD effect is greatly enhanced at 3 T, leading to greater confidence and accuracy when performing fMRI studies.

Although chemical shift increases with field strength, the impact of misregistration artifact can be reduced by use of increased receiver bandwidths compared with lower fields. With MR spectroscopy, the increase in chemical shift provides the ability to achieve increased spectral resolution—making it possible to resolve metabolites with relatively small variations in frequency—and the increase in SNR makes possible shorter scans and smaller voxels.

In summary, the introduction of 3 T systems into the clinical environment has presented many challenges. However, with optimization of hardware and imaging protocols, spectacular results can be achieved that are simply not possible at lower fields. It is clear that 3 T represents the new mainstream high-end clinical imaging field strength for MR.

William H. Faulkner Jr., B.S., R.T. (R) (MR) (CT), F.S.M.R.T.
Director of Education
Chattanooga Imaging
CEO
William Faulkner & Associates
Chattanooga, Tennessee

Preface

The objective of this textbook is to present practical, important concepts relevant to clinical MR at 3 T, focusing on images and clinical results. Differences from diagnostic studies at 1.5 T are emphasized. Recommendations are made for optimization of imaging technique at 3 T to assure high image quality.

The text is organized into concise chapters, each discussing an important point relevant to clinical 3 T MR and illustrated with images from routine patient exams. The topics covered encompass the breadth of the field, from imaging basics and pulse sequences to advanced topics including diffusion tensor imaging, arterial spin-labeling, susceptibility-weighted imaging, and spectroscopy. Following a discussion of the physics of 3 T that emphasizes SAR and safety issues, the text proceeds with an in-depth look at imaging of the body organized by anatomic region. A large section is devoted to clinical imaging of the head and spine, with the text then proceeding to the musculoskeletal system, followed by imaging of the heart, continuing with studies of the abdomen and pelvis, and concluding with contrast-enhanced MRA. Discussion of the latest hardware and software developments, from parallel imaging and multichannel technology to low SAR techniques, is integrated throughout the text as these topics are critical to imaging at 3 T.

3 T MR represents a major forefront of diagnostic radiology today. Heat deposition, changes in T1 relaxation rates, susceptibility differences, and possible increased sensitivity to motion artifacts represent challenges to clinical implementation, which have already largely been overcome. The situation appears remarkably similar to that encountered more than 15 years ago as the field of magnetic resonance transitioned from what was then low and mid-field to 1.5 T. Current generation 3 T MR units already provide markedly improved imaging versus 1.5 T in the vast majority of clinical exams. A common dilemma due to the available SNR is the choice between a "long" very high resolution scan and a fast, lower resolution study. The sophistication of the technique and continued advances dictate that magnetic resonance, as the field transitions from 1.5 to 3 T, will continue to play a dominant role in clinical medicine for the foreseeable future.

Val M. Runge, M.D.
Editor-in-Chief, Investigative Radiology
Robert and Alma Moreton Centennial Chair in Radiology
Scott & White Clinic and Hospital
Texas A&M Health Science Center
Temple, Texas

Contributors

Jonmenjoy Biswas, M.D.
Department of Radiology
Scott & White Clinic and Hospital
Texas A&M Health Science Center
Temple, Texas

Andreas Boss, M.D.
Department of Diagnostic Radiology
Section on Experimental Radiology
University Hospital of Tübingen
Tübingen, Germany

Robert S. Case, M.D.
Department of Radiology
Scott & White Clinic and Hospital
Texas A&M Health Science Center
Temple, Texas

Ethan A. Colby, M.D.
Department of Radiology
Scott & White Clinic and Hospital
Texas A&M Health Science Center
Temple, Texas

**William H. Faulkner Jr., B.S.,
R.T.(R)(MR)(CT), F.S.M.R.T.**
Director of Education
Chattanooga Imaging
CEO
William Faulkner & Associates
Chattanooga, Tennessee

Jurgen J. Fütterer, M.D., Ph.D.
Department of Radiology
Radboud University Nijmegen Medical Center
Nijmegen, The Netherlands

Elizabeth M. Hecht, M.D.
Clinical Assistant Professor
Department of Radiology
New York University Medical Center
New York, New York

Benjamin Hyman, M.D.
Department of Radiology
Scott & White Clinic and Hospital
Texas A&M Health Science Center
Temple, Texas

Harald Kramer, M.D.
Department of Clinical Radiology
University Hospitals-Grosshadern
Ludwig-Maximilians-University Munich
Munich, Germany

Petros Martirosian, M.Sc.
Section on Experimental Radiology
University Hospital of Tübingen
Tübingen, Germany

Elmar M. Merkle, M.D.
Professor of Radiology
Director of Body MR Imaging
Duke University Medical Center
Durham, North Carolina

Henrik J. Michaely, M.D.
Department of Clinical Radiology
University Hospitals-Grosshadern
Ludwig-Maximilians-University Munich
Munich, Germany

Wolfgang R. Nitz, Ph.D.
Senior Application Scientist
MR Division
Siemens Medical Solutions
Erlangen, Germany

John T. Pitts, R.T.(R)(MR)
Manager of Applications and Technical
    Marketing, Eastern Division
Invivo Diagnostic Imaging
Pewaukee, Wisconsin

Val M. Runge, M.D.
Robert and Alma Moreton Centennial
    Chair in Radiology
Department of Radiology
Scott & White Clinic and Hospital
Texas A&M Health Science Center
Temple, Texas

Richard K. Sanders, M.D.
Assistant Professor of Radiology
Department of Radiology, MSK Division
University of Utah Health Sciences Center
Salt Lake City, Utah

Tom W.J. Scheenen, Ph.D.
MR Physicist
Department of Radiology
Radboud University Nijmegen Medical Center
Nijmegen, The Netherlands

Fritz Schick, M.D., Ph.D.
Professor of Experimental Radiology
Department of Diagnostic Radiology
Section on Experimental Radiology
University Hospital of Tübingen
Tübingen, Germany

Stuart H. Schmeets, B.S., R.T. (R)(MR)
Advanced Specialist Ultra High-Field
    MRI Applications
Siemens Medical Solutions USA, Inc.
Malvern, Pennsylvania

Mitchell D. Schnall, M.D., Ph.D.
Professor
Department of Radiology
University of Pennsylvania School
    of Medicine
Philadelphia, Pennsylvania

Stefan O. Schoenberg, M.D.
Associate Professor of Radiology
Associate Chair of Clinical Operations
Department of Clinical Radiology
University Hospitals-Grosshadern
Ludwig-Maximilians-University Munich
Munich, Germany

Harold L. Sonnier, M.D.
Chief Resident
Department of Radiology
Scott & White Clinic and Hospital
Texas A&M Health Science Center
Temple, Texas

Satoru Takahashi, M.D., Ph.D.
Department of Radiology
Radboud University Nijmegen Medical
    Center
Nijmegen, The Netherlands

Bernd J. Wintersperger, M.D.
Department of Clinical Radiology
University Hospitals-Grosshadern
Ludwig-Maximilians-University Munich
Munich, Germany

Ronald L. Wolf, M.D., Ph.D.
Assistant Professor
Department of Radiology
Neuroradiology Section
University of Pennsylvania School of
    Medicine
Hospital of the University of Pennsylvania
Philadelphia, Pennsylvania

Christoph J. Zech, M.D.
Department of Clinical Radiology
University Hospitals-Grosshadern
Ludwig-Maximilians-University Munich
Munich, Germany

Robert A. Zimmerman, M.D.
Professor
Department of Radiology
University of Pennsylvania School of
    Medicine
Children's Hospital of Philadelphia
Philadelphia, Pennsylvania

1 Basic Principles of MR
Wolfgang R. Nitz

If you expose a patient inside a magnetic field to a relatively weak electromagnetic radio-frequency (RF) field, the patient's body will respond by emitting a very small but detectable electromagnetic RF signal itself. A quantum mechanical property termed *nuclear spin* is the cause of this phenomenon. This property will only show up in the presence of a strong magnetic field. The nucleus itself behaves like it has an angular momentum correlated with a magnetic moment—this behavior is termed *nuclear spin*. As a quantum mechanical property, the spin of a hydrogen atom nucleus is allowed to align itself either parallel or antiparallel to the direction of the magnetic field, as illustrated in **Fig. 1–1A**, which also shows the common visualization of the two different energy levels of these nuclei. Although a parallel alignment is the preferred status of the lowest energy level, nature provides only limited seats, and the remaining spins not getting a seat have to accept the antiparallel alignment. Quantum mechanics postulates parallel or antiparallel alignment with no other choice. The energy difference between these two levels can be expressed, according to Einstein, by the frequency of an electromagnetic field. The magnetic field strength is measured in tesla (T), and for a 1.5 T system, the energy difference of the two levels corresponds with an RF field of 63 MHz. For a 3 T system, that

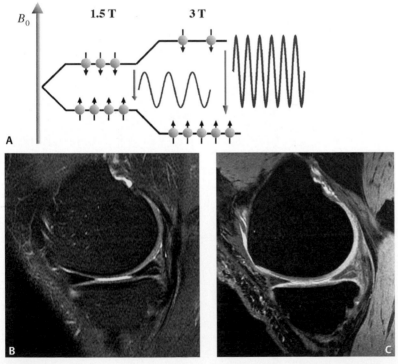

Figure 1–1

energy difference doubles to 126 MHz, and to make things more attractive, in that case more seats are available for the low-energy position. The mechanism to get the patient's body to emit an RF signal is to move some of the parallel-aligned spins to a higher energy level, the antiparallel alignment. To do so, the frequency of the transmitted RF field has to match the frequency given by the energy difference (i.e., the transmitted frequency has to be in "resonance" with what is also called the Larmor frequency). After "exciting" the spins, they will, within milliseconds, fall back into their old positions, emitting the energy difference as RF signal, also called the MR signal. Whereas the energy difference is reflected via the Larmor frequency, the intensity or signal strength depends on how many "seats" can be traded. Generally speaking, signal strength scales with field strength. The higher the field strength, the stronger the MR signal will be. A meniscal tear is demonstrated on a 3-mm slice acquired using a 1.5 T system **(Fig. 1–1B)** adjacent to a comparable 1.5-mm slice acquired on a 3 T system **(Fig. 1–1C)**. Due to the greater available signal strength on the higher field system (3 T), a thinner slice thickness is clinically feasible and can be employed for improved diagnosis.

The fascinating part of magnetic resonance is the fact that the whole body experiences the RF pulse, but only those areas in resonance with the frequency content of the pulse will get excited. Altering the magnetic field strength locally with a magnetic field gradient (GS) prior to sending the RF pulse will allow a slice-selective excitation. When moving back to the lower energy level, the nuclei will emit the energy difference in the form of an MR signal. The frequency of the MR signal is given by the current local magnetic field strength at the time of the emission. Applying local magnetic field gradients (GR) during readout of the data will provide a frequency spectrum of the MR signal that contains spatial information.

◆ Why 3 T?

The measurement time in MR imaging is given by the time needed to fill k-space. In conventional spin-echo imaging, as illustrated in **Figs. 1–2A** and **1–2B,** this is the number of phase-encoding steps multiplied by the repetition time and the number of excitations. The measurement time is significantly reduced when using multiple phase-encoded spin echoes as done with fast spin-echo (FSE) imaging. However, this

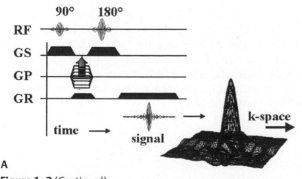

A

Figure 1–2 (*Continued*)

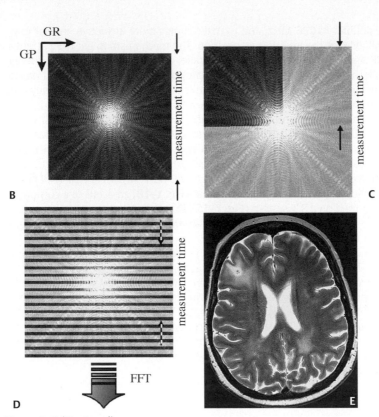

GR
GP

measurement time

measurement time

B

C

measurement time

FFT

D

E

Figure 1–2 (*Continued*)

is only effective in proton density- and T2-weighted imaging. In half-Fourier imaging, advantage is taken of the fact that k-space is symmetric **(Fig. 1–2C)**. Measurement time is reduced at the expense of the signal-to-noise ratio (SNR) by measuring only half of k-space. Skipping every other Fourier line **(Fig. 1–2D)** will reduce measurement time by a factor of two, but, as this step is identical to a smaller field of view in the phase-encoding direction, it will lead to significant wraparound artifacts and reduced SNR. Wraparound artifacts can, however, be eliminated by using the spatial informa-tion provided by coil elements distributed in the phase-encoding direction (parallel imaging). What remains is the drop in SNR. The signal gain in high-field imaging, in moving from 1.5 to 3 T, seems to offer the solution. **Figure 1–2E** presents an image from a patient with a right frontal metastatic lesion. Measurement time for this T2-weighted FSE scan was 44 sec for 32 slices with a slice thickness of 3 mm and a matrix size of 269×512 utilizing parallel imaging; this case shows the reduction in scan time that can be achieved at 3 T due to the available SNR.

2 Components of an MR Scanner

Wolfgang R. Nitz

◆ The Magnet

As previously stated, to see the nuclear spin phenomenon, a strong magnetic field is required. The field strength is expressed in tesla. The earth field has ~0.00005 T. The magnet keeping the refrigerator door closed has ~0.005 T. If you were to glue ~16 tons of permanent magnets together, a field strength of 0.35 T can be achieved. To achieve a higher field strength, the phenomenon of superconductivity has to be used. Superconductivity is again a quantum mechanical property that results in the ability to conduct electricity without the loss of energy. Certain alloys display superconductivity at cryogenic temperatures (placed in a bath of liquid helium [4.2 kelvin = −269°Celsius = −452°Fahrenheit]). The field strength is "simply" the product of the number of windings and the current driven through the coil. Because the current amplitude is close to the limit, going from 1.5 T to 3 T will require additional coil windings to increase the field strength, making the magnet heavier and more expensive.

◆ The Transmitting Radio-Frequency Coil

As outlined previously, to "excite the spins," energy needs to be transferred into the patient using RF with a frequency identical to the Larmor frequency of the protons within water or fat-bound hydrogen atoms located in the region to be imaged. It is very cumbersome to discuss excitation and refocusing on a quantum mechanical level. Fortunately, a huge number of quantum mechanical properties (specifically, the spin properties of the significant number of protons within a single voxel) can be dealt with using classical physics. It is valid to just consider the net magnetization that is building up due to the imbalance between parallel- and antiparallel-aligned nuclear spins. That magnetization is building up in the longitudinal direction, is behaving like a rotating magnet, and is tilted by the excitation pulse 90 degrees into a so-called transverse plane. The magnetic field component B_1 of the RF pulse is responsible for the tilting. The tilting will only succeed for the magnetization precessing with the same frequency as the rotating B_1 field. This is the magic behind slice-selective excitation. Engineering of the transmitter coil for a 3 T system is not much different than that for a 1.5 T system, except for doubling of the resonance frequency. An important factor for the transmitter coil design at 3 T is to reduce the RF field experienced by the patient to the smallest region possible. The specific absorption rate (SAR) is the energy per unit time deposited into the patient, potentially causing an increase in body temperature. The effect is a function of the effective RF volume the patient experiences.

◆ The Gradients

To locally manipulate the magnetic field for the purpose of preparing a slice-selective excitation or spatial encoding of the MR signal, a frame of copper windings is inserted inside the magnet. The currents sent through these copper windings will diminish the field on one end and enhance the field on the other end for a user-defined direction. There are three physical directions of these so-called gradient coils (x, y, and z), but they can be combined to produce a linear magnetic field gradient in any direction. The strength of a gradient coil is measured in mT/m, and a common benchmark is 40 mT/m. The time necessary to reach the maximum amplitude in combination with the value of that maximum defines the slew rate of the gradient system. A state-of-the-art value is 200 $T \cdot m^{-1} \cdot s^{-1}$. The gradient strength is not correlated with the field strength of the system. However, one does have to take into account that there are additional mechanical (Lorentz) forces on the gradient system in the presence of a stronger magnetic field. The Lorentz force describes the mechanical burden on a wire that carries an electric current within a magnetic field. Because 3 T presents a stronger field as compared with a 1.5 T system, increased mechanical forces will cause a stronger vibration of the gradient coil. Without counteracting measures, one would thus expect a 3 T system to produce a stronger acoustic noise than a 1.5 T system. **Figure 2–1** illustrates the gradient coil hidden behind the inside covers of the magnet, with the transmitting RF coil inserted into the gradient coil.

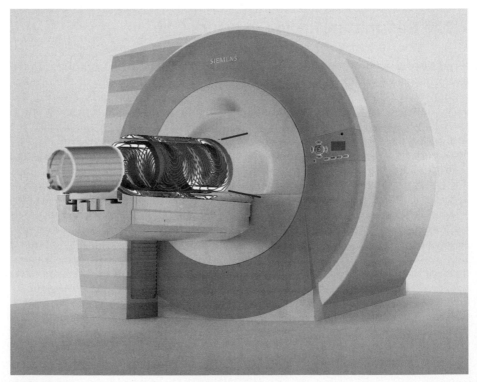

Figure 2–1

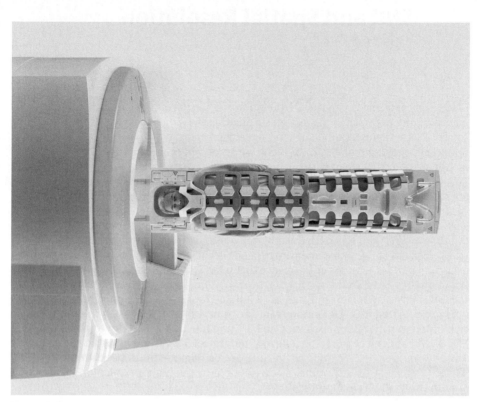

Figure 2–2

◆ The Imaging Matrix

In a worst-case scenario, one can use the transmitter coil to receive the MR signal. But it is a great advantage to have the receiver coil as close as possible to the source of the signal, which is usually done with dedicated surface coils. The term *imaging matrix* has been introduced to describe a large number of coil elements covering a specific anatomic region **(Fig. 2–2)**. Small coils are beneficial for good SNR. Several small coils ensure sufficient coverage, and the spatial distribution of coil elements can be used to retrieve spatial information that otherwise would have to be measured. Because all these coil or matrix elements are measuring the signal parallel to one another, the term *parallel imaging* has been established. Parallel imaging will be discussed later as a potential method to reduce the power deposition into a patient.

3 SNR and Spatial Resolution

Wolfgang R. Nitz

Diagnostic confidence in image interpretation is a function of the ratio between the signal intensity from the voxel in the excited slice within the patient's body and the underlying "noise." Noise represents the sudden appearance and the fast vanishing of detected or mimicked amplitudes of electromagnetic waves of significant amplitude that show up as an MR signal. For all sources, the patient's body is considered the major source of noise. That is why surface coils, which only see a limited region and therefore pick up less noise, are recommended in MR imaging. The noise can be assumed to be equally spread across the frequency range of our imaging protocol. Because frequency encoding is used to extract spatial information, and two adjacent voxels are defined as having a difference in frequency of a few hertz (also called bandwidth), the noise contribution will be less for low-bandwidth sequences. The signal intensity depends on how many protons are involved in the excitation process, with the consequence that if the voxel is bigger, the higher is the number of protons and thus the stronger is the signal. The larger the field strength, the larger the ratio between parallel- and antiparallel-aligned spins and the stronger the signal.

Figures 3–1A and **3–1B** demonstrate the appearance of a vascular malformation in two different patients, one scanned at 1.5 T and one at 3 T. The T1-weighted image in **Fig. 3–1A** has been acquired on a new-generation 1.5 T system using an FSE sequence with a scan time of 2:42 min:sec. In comparison, **Fig. 3–1B** has been acquired within 47 sec (a much faster scan time, made possible by the higher available SNR) on a 3 T system using a T1-FLAIR. protocol.

◆ Slice Thickness

The voxel size is a linear function of slice thickness and so also is SNR. The thinner the slice, the better the spatial resolution and the less the partial volume effect, with a linear drop in SNR as a trade-off.

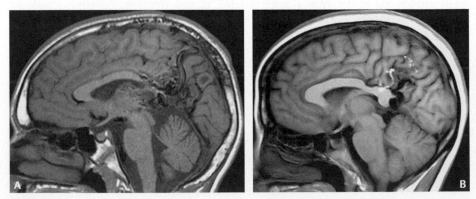

Figure 3–1

◆ Field of View

The voxel size is the product of slice thickness, dimension in the direction of phase encoding, and dimension in the direction of frequency encoding. Reducing the field of view (FOV) will reduce the dimension in frequency as well as phase-encoding direction. The voxel size and the correlated signal intensity will drop with the power of two for any FOV reduction. The smaller the voxel, the better the spatial resolution. Partial volume effects and susceptibility artifacts are reduced with increased spatial resolution. A reduction in voxel size, however, leads to a loss in SNR. This loss is a linear function of the voxel volume.

◆ Rectangular Field of View

The historic main purpose of a rectangular field of view (RecFOV) was to reduce measurement time while keeping spatial resolution constant. Keeping in perspective that each received signal is the sum of all individual signals from each voxel, each acquisition, whether it is phase encoded or not, will contribute to a better SNR. Reducing the FOV in the direction of phase encoding while maintaining spatial resolution (e.g., number of phase-encoding steps goes from 256 to 128) will reduce the measurement time by a factor of two and will lead to a drop in SNR down to 0.71 ($1/\sqrt{2}$).

◆ Matrix Size

The base matrix size considers the number of columns and rows to be equal. A drop in matrix size by a factor of two will decrease the spatial resolution by increasing the voxel size by a factor of four (2×2). As each phase-encoding step is also considered an additional acquisition, the fourfold signal gain is to be multiplied by 0.71 ($1/\sqrt{2}$). Dropping the matrix size by a factor of two will reduce the measurement time by a factor of two and will lead to a gain in SNR by a factor of 2.84 ($2 \times 2/\sqrt{2}$) at the expense of spatial resolution (increased partial volume effects and susceptibility artifacts).

4 SNR and k-space
Wolfgang R. Nitz

The scan (or measurement) time is dictated by the number of Fourier lines to be acquired, also called the number of phase-encoding steps or k-space lines. Measurement time can be decreased by reducing the number of Fourier lines. Reducing the phase resolution will cut down the measurement time and also lead to an increase in SNR, though at the expense of spatial resolution in the direction of phase encoding. The latter typically causes more prominent truncation artifacts within the image. Increasing the number of Fourier lines while keeping the spatial resolution constant is called phase oversampling, which will eliminate wraparound artifacts and also lead to a gain in SNR due to the additional measurements, though at the expense of measurement time. Taking advantage of the k-space symmetry, it is possible to retrospectively reconstruct the other half of k-space, which will lead to a reduction in measurement time, though at the expense of SNR.

◆ The Phase Resolution

The phase resolution indicates the spatial asymmetry in the direction of phase encoding with respect to the base matrix size. An alternative to reduce measurement time is to reduce the number of phase-encoding steps, at the expense of spatial resolution in the direction of phase encoding. As a consequence, the voxel size increases in the direction of phase encoding, and more protons will contribute to the signal that is identified to be coming out of the single voxel. Moving from a 100% resolution to a 50% resolution will cause the voxel to increase in size by a factor of two, and one would expect the signal to increase by the same amount. Because each measured phase-encoding line contributes to the SNR, and those lines are now reduced by a factor of two, the gain in SNR has to be divided by $\sqrt{2}$. Reducing the measurement time by a factor of two while decreasing the spatial resolution in the direction of phase encoding by a factor of two when moving from a 100% phase resolution to 50% will thus lead to a gain in SNR by a factor of $2/\sqrt{2} = \sqrt{2} = 1.41$.

◆ Phase Oversampling

The system will select a sampling grid according to the base matrix size and the phase resolution. Higher frequencies outside the FOV will be sampled as if they appear within the FOV leading to wraparound artifacts. One way to eliminate these artifacts is to "oversample." That step is equivalent to still showing the same FOV but increasing the "measured" FOV. There is no penalty in doubling the number of sampling points in the direction of frequency encoding, and this is commonly implemented as default with no option to deselect. In the direction of phase encoding, additional sampling points represent the measurement of additional Fourier lines

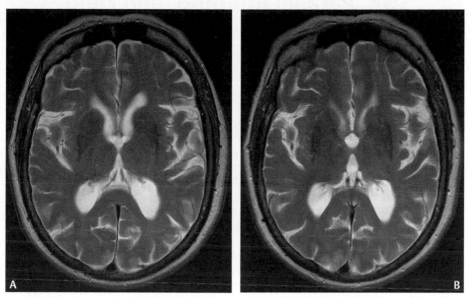

Figure 4–1

and will lead to an increase in measurement time. As each measured Fourier line contributes to the overall SNR, phase oversampling will not only eliminate wraparound artifacts but will also lead to an SNR gain. Selecting a 100% phase oversampling will double the measurement time, will double the measured FOV, and will lead to an increase in SNR by a factor of $\sqrt{2} = 1.41$

◆ Partial Fourier

In theory, k-space shows Hermetian symmetry, and it should be sufficient to measure only one quadrant. In practice, phase distortions destroy that symmetry, and to eliminate the related artifacts, commonly all of k-space is measured. Partial Fourier is an approach to skip the measurement of certain parts of k-space, mirroring the missing lines from the other half of the measured k-space. Because each measured phase-encoding line contributes to the SNR, and those lines are now reduced by a factor of two, the loss in SNR is $1/\sqrt{2} = 0.71$ (with a half-Fourier acquisition). **Figure 4–1A** has been acquired using a 512 matrix and partial Fourier imaging to achieve a measurement time of 1:44 minutes. **Figure 4–1B** has been acquired in 1:07 minutes using a minor asymmetry of the matrix size (211 × 512). SNR is improved in **Fig. 4–1B** due to the sacrifice in spatial resolution, with a shorter measurement time being an additional advantage.

5 SNR, Parallel Imaging, and Field Strength

Wolfgang R. Nitz

Surface coils have been used from the very beginning of MR to gain SNR by getting closer to the origin of the signal. It turned out that in making coil dimensions small, there is a substantial gain in SNR. To achieve sufficient anatomic coverage, multiple small coils are used, the latter termed *coil arrays* or *imaging matrixes*. It did not take long to discover that the spatial distribution of these coil elements could be used to derive spatial information, allowing a reduction of the number of k-space lines to be measured without sacrificing spatial resolution. Reducing measurement time while maintaining the spatial resolution usually comes at the expense of SNR. Gaining SNR by using higher-field systems like 3 T will provide the flexibility to take advantage of shortening measurement time by employing parallel imaging. *Parallel imaging* is the general expression for using multiple coil elements to derive spatial information, as all these coils are measuring the signal at the same time (in "parallel").

◆ Surface Coils

It is beneficial for overall SNR to get as close as possible to the origin of the signal. Receiving coils that are mounted on the surface of the patient's body have been termed *surface coils*. With the introduction of multiple separate RF receiver channels and the use of a significant number of coil elements, the term *imaging matrix* has been introduced. The SNR gain is a function of the matrix design and is dependent on the distance between the signal source and the next matrix element.

◆ Parallel Imaging, mSENSE or GRAPPA

By using image matrixes with matrix elements distributed in the direction of phase encoding, it is possible to skip the measurement of Fourier lines and use the spatial information of the distributed matrix elements in that direction instead. As there are fewer Fourier lines acquired, there will be a decrease in SNR. If an acceleration factor of two is selected, the measurement of every second Fourier line will be skipped and the measurement time will be reduced by a factor of two with no penalty in spatial resolution. Because the number of Fourier lines is now reduced by a factor of two, the loss in SNR is $1/\sqrt{2} = 0.71$.

◆ Field Strength

With an increase in field strength, it is not only the energy difference between parallel- and antiparallel-aligned spins that is increased but also the difference in the number of spins that are going to be moved to a higher level and then fall back into the

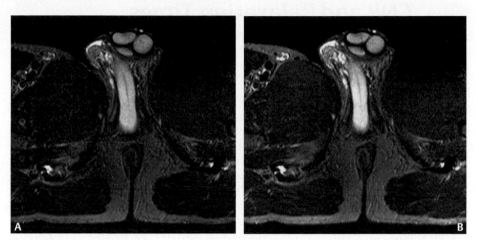

Figure 5–1

old position while emitting a strong signal. The gain in signal is proportional to the increase in field strength. That gain can be used to either shorten measurement time or increase spatial resolution, with one approach (for the latter) being use of the aforementioned "parallel imaging" technique. Axial STIR images were acquired on a male patient (soccer player) complaining about groin pain. **Figure 5–1** demonstrates a small fluid collection consistent with osteitis pubis, or inflammation of the symphysis pubis, which is commonly seen in soccer players. **Figure 5–1A** was acquired using one acquisition and no parallel imaging. **Figure 5–1B** was acquired using two acquisitions utilizing a parallel acquisition technique (PAT) factor of 2 to keep the measurement time constant.

♦ Bandwidth

To identify the location of the signal, magnetic field gradients are used to cause a local dependence of the Larmor frequencies. It is incumbent upon the user to select, per definition, the difference in frequency between adjacent voxels. That difference is termed the (frequency) *bandwidth*. Unused frequencies are cut off with a filter, and only the frequency noise within the image bandwidth will contribute to the overall noise level. Image noise is reduced by using a low-bandwidth protocol. The noise is proportional to $\sqrt{v}$, with v being the bandwidth of the protocol. The length of the data acquisition window is given by the time needed to allow a 360-degree turn of the transverse magnetization for the adjacent voxel. That will take longer for a low-bandwidth sequence leading to a prolonged data acquisition window resulting in longer echo times, making the protocol more sensitive to flow, motion, and susceptibility artifacts. Because the chemical shift artifact increases with field strength, a higher imaging bandwidth is typically required at 3 T to reduce that artifact. The use of a higher bandwidth will lead to a reduction in SNR, diminishing the SNR gain correlated with higher field strength.

6 CNR and Relaxation Times

Wolfgang R. Nitz

To identify normal and abnormal tissue structures with any imaging modality, a difference in signal intensity between the abnormality and the surrounding normal tissue is necessary. To identify small objects, it is essential that the signal difference exceeds the image noise level. The ratio between the signal difference of two different tissues and the noise is called the contrast-to-noise ratio (CNR). Because it is difficult to distinguish between signal variations due to structural changes within the same tissue and the true image noise, the standard deviation of the signal in the background (typically air) is commonly taken to calculate the CNR.

The general signal contribution assigned to a single voxel has been discussed in the previous case. There are three main tissue-specific factors that may cause a difference in signal intensity in MR. These include proton density, T1 relaxation, and T2 relaxation. The influence of these tissue-specific parameters on image contrast is dictated by the type of imaging sequence used and the selected protocol parameters. The contrast on an image is termed accordingly *proton density–weighted*, *T1-weighted*, or *T2-weighted*.

The proton density of the tissue is not influenced by the field strength and therefore does not need to be discussed further. The T1-relaxation time describes the temporal course of the recovery of the longitudinal magnetization after excitation. This tissue-specific T1-relaxation time is a function of the molecular motion. To relax after excitation, the excited spins have to experience field fluctuations close to their Larmor frequency to transfer the energy to the environment (spin-lattice interaction). While molecular motion is of course not a function of field strength, the Larmor frequency is. Because the Larmor frequency is significantly increased in going from 1.5 T to 3 T, the spin-lattice interaction is hampered, leading to prolonged T1-relaxation times. The protocol parameters to achieve T1-weighted images at 3 T have to be adapted accordingly compared with parameters used on 1.5 T systems.

In general, T2 values are unrelated to field strength. T2-relaxation time is solely a function of molecular motion as the adjacent proton within the same molecule is imposing its magnetic moment upon its neighbor, causing a field increase or field decrease on a molecular level depending on the orientation of the molecule relative to the magnetic field. For a rapidly tumbling free water molecule, the averaging effect will counterbalance all interactions, leading to relatively slow signal decay due to rapid changes in spin-spin interaction (long T2-relaxation time). However, the situation changes in the presence of tissue iron; for example, hemosiderin (the presence of which seems to shorten T2-relaxation times but is indeed a T2* effect combined with the diffusion of water molecules in between excitation and refocusing pulses). These apparent T2 changes are related to magnetic field strength and are not as prominent at lower fields. Imaging at 3 T may thus contribute further to the understanding of neurodegenerative conditions that involve altered brain iron levels, due to the greater

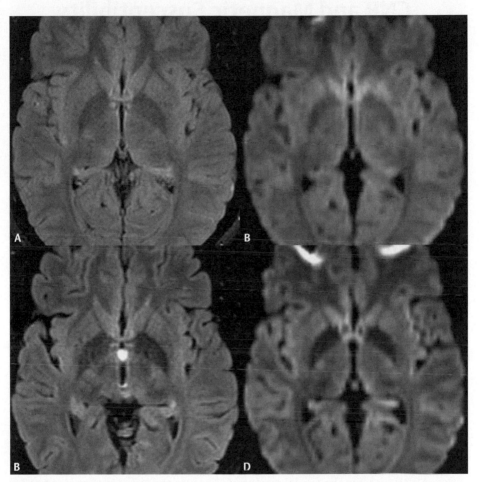

Figure 6–1

effect at higher field strength of iron on T2. Illustrated in **Fig. 6–1** are **(A, C)** FLAIR and **(B, D)** diffusion-weighted scans at **(A, B)** 1.5 and **(C, D)** 3 T obtained in the same patient. Note the change in tissue contrast with increasing field, best seen in the basal ganglia. The globus pallidus is of strikingly lower signal intensity at 3 T relative to the caudate and putamen, due to the effect of iron, with a similar but less evident effect in normal white matter (best seen on the diffusion-weighted scans). In addition to the three main tissue-specific parameters (proton density, T1, and T2), there are a variety of other factors in MR, including magnetic susceptibility, T2*, diffusion, perfusion, flow, magnetization transfer, and tissue elasticity that can be used to alter image contrast.

7 CNR and Magnetic Susceptibility
Wolfgang R. Nitz

The magnetic susceptibility is the degree of magnetization that a material, or tissue, exhibits in response to a magnetic field and should not be confused with the nuclear magnetization caused by the nuclear spins. Material that diminishes the magnetic field is called diamagnetic. Material enhancing the magnetic field up to 1% is called paramagnetic, and material that enhances the field by more than 1% and keeps a degree of magnetization once the external field vanishes is called ferromagnetic. Differences in magnetic susceptibility are also referred to as susceptibility gradients. Tissue boundaries within a patient are the origin of local magnetic field inhomogeneities due to differences in magnetic susceptibility. Local changes in the magnetic field strength will cause differences in Larmor frequencies, leading to a rapid signal dephasing. Because the magnetic susceptibility is usually not a function of field strength (with the exception of ferromagnetic material), the difference in Larmor frequencies scales with the strength of the external magnetic field. As a consequence, susceptibility-related artifacts are more prominent at 3 T than they are at 1.5 T. This can be both an advantage as well as a disadvantage. The majority of biological tissue is slightly diamagnetic; that is, the magnetic field inside the tissue is diminished by less than 1%. The magnetic susceptibility of deoxyhemoglobin is paramagnetic, leading to a decrease in diamagnetism for deoxygenated blood as compared with oxygenated blood. The signal in regions with oxyhemoglobin shows a slightly stronger signal than in regions with deoxyhemoglobin. This has been termed *BOLD* (blood oxygenation level dependent) contrast and is used in functional imaging. Because susceptibility-related effects are more prominent with higher field strength, the BOLD effect will be enhanced at 3 T as compared with 1.5 T. Addressing a potential disadvantage for 3 T, the signal void related to susceptibility artifacts (which are more prominent at 3 T) is a function of the frequency distribution within a single voxel. Susceptibility artifacts can thus be reduced by increasing the spatial resolution. Because the latter is often done at 3 T, to take advantage of the additional SNR, the reduction of susceptibility artifacts is addressed as well. **Figure 7–1** illustrates the effect of susceptibility gradients close to the orbital region for two patients with different cerebral malignancies using diffusion-weighted echo planar imaging: **(A)** and **(C)**, in a patient with an astrocytoma, were acquired at 1.5 T with b-values of zero and 1000, respectively; **(B)** and **(D)**, in a patient with an ependymoma, were acquired at 3 T with b-values of zero and 1000. The spatial resolution of the scans at 1.5 and 3 T was held constant. Note the greater magnitude of the susceptibility artifact anteriorly (arrows), originating from the orbits, in the images at 3 T.

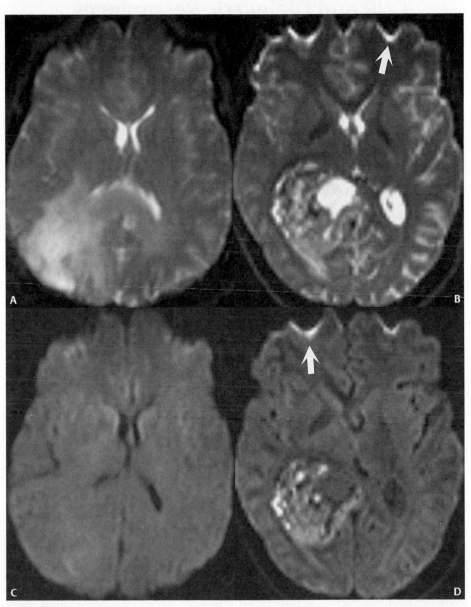

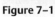
Figure 7–1

8 CNR and Dielectric Resonances

Wolfgang R. Nitz

Several factors contribute to changes in the signal amplitude within the FOV for otherwise identical tissue. The two main factors are coil design and B_1 field inhomogeneities.

◆ Coil Design

For parallel imaging, it is desired to have a confined sensitivity profile for each matrix element. This will help in identifying wraparound artifacts in parallel imaging. The latter uses the spatial distribution of coil elements, allowing some phase-encoding measurements to be skipped. It will be beneficial for the overall SNR if all coil elements represent each location with the same signal intensity. Algorithms using distributed coil elements to retrieve spatial information require distinguished sensitivity profiles for each coil element. Sophisticated coil design uses mode switching to either arrange matrix coil elements to produce maximum SNR and an optimized homogeneous sensitivity profile or to switch to multiple RF channels using the different coil-sensitivity profiles to allow parallel imaging.

◆ B_1 Field Inhomogeneities

The patient's body presents a dielectric medium that will attenuate the electric and magnetic field components of a propagating electromagnetic wave, whether it is the transmitted RF or the emitted MR signal. For the RF wavelength of a 1.5 T system, this effect is almost negligible. For the RF wavelength within the patient's body at 3 T, it poses a serious challenge. A somewhat comparable limit is present in ultrasound, where it is well known that higher ultrasound frequencies are prohibitive for the evaluation of structures located deeper in the patient's body. For MR imaging, that situation is less dramatic, although noticeable. An additional concern is the reflection of electromagnetic waves at tissue boundaries with different conductivities (e.g., body to air). As the wavelength of the RF field inside the patient's body becomes comparable with a human-sized sample, the concern has been that this will lead to a standing-wave behavior also referred to as dielectric resonance. Fortunately, the standing-wave pattern and associated dielectric resonances documented in pure water samples cannot be sustained in the human body because of the strong decay of the RF electromagnetic wave caused by sample resistance. The remaining concern is solely the exponential RF field attenuation within the patient that varies with depth from the skin.

◆ Normalization

Similar to the time gain compensation amplification used in ultrasound, a normalization filter can be applied to eliminate or at least reduce the signal inhomogeneity caused by the aforementioned phenomenon. Conventional normalization filters solely rely on image information. A more sophisticated normalization filter uses prescan information to identify in advance the signal distribution as a function of B_1 field inhomogeneity and coil-sensitivity profile. The resultant image appears more homogeneous as a result of using any of these normalization algorithms, with one drawback being that the noise in areas with originally low signal intensities will also be enhanced. The normalization filter will only mask the spatially varying CNR. The benefits for the overall CNR gain in using the aforementioned coil design outweigh the disadvantages of having to normalize the images. **Figure 8–1** presents images of an axial postcontrast T1-weighted gradient-echo (GRE) imaging scan in a postoperative astrocytoma (residual, small, enhancing tumor nodules are noted at the edges of the surgical bed, see arrows). **Figure 8–1A** demonstrates the combined effect of the sensitivity profiles of the multiple coil elements surrounding the head and the B_1 field inhomogeneity. **Figure 8–1B** has been acquired using the same protocol with the exception of the use of a normalization filter during image reconstruction.

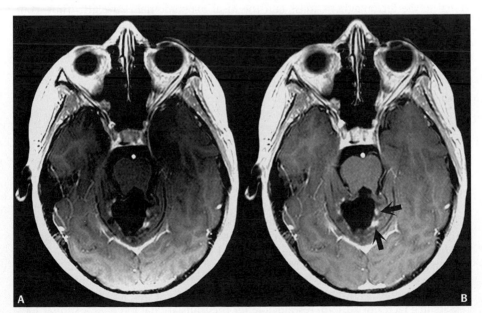

Figure 8–1

9 Torque and Attraction
Wolfgang R. Nitz

It is well-known, and an important safety consideration for clinical MR, that a strong magnetic field will pull any ferromagnetic object into the magnet and will twist any ferromagnetic aneurysm clip. Despite educational efforts in this area, there have been several fatal injuries due to misunderstandings, miscommunication, and underestimation of the underlying power that a magnetic field exerts.

◆ Torque

Exposing a ferromagnetic object to a magnetic field will cause the object to become magnetized, which is to become a magnetic dipole. If the ferromagnetic object is symmetric and if the magnetic field is homogeneous, nothing will happen. For example, a ferromagnetic ball, once in the center of the magnet, will not experience any further forces. If the ferromagnetic object is asymmetric, like a ferromagnetic rod or a pair of scissors, the object will experience a significant torque, which is proportional to the magnetic field strength and the magnetic moment of the object. The latter is proportional to the ferromagnetic mass and the local magnetic field strength. Thus, compared with a 1.5 T system, the torque experienced on a 3 T system "simply" increases by a factor of four. This torque will be greatest near the magnet center. Needle-shaped objects will tend to turn their long axis parallel to the field direction, and plate-like objects will tend to turn their flat surfaces parallel to the field lines. In many situations, the torque represents a greater hazard than the translational force.

◆ Attractive Forces

Ferromagnetic objects with very large magnetic susceptibilities tend to become magnetized in a strong external magnetic field, and they will be pulled to the location where the magnetic field is at its maximum. In a first approximation, the magnetization of the ferromagnetic object is proportional to the local field strength. The translational force depends on the fringe field distribution and the field strength. Illustrated in **Fig. 9–1** for a 3 T magnet is the fringe field distribution for the longitudinal axes (which are symmetric) and one lateral direction. For the magnet illustrated, the maximum spatial gradient of B_0 is 7 T/m at the inside of the bore ~80 cm from the isocenter of the magnet. Multiplied by the local magnetic field at that location (2.78 T), this results in a factor of 20 T^2/m responsible for the translational force. At a similar location with a 1.5 T system, one will find a force of 6 T^2/m. In this example, the translational force will approximately triple for a 3 T system compared with a 1.5 T system. Once the ferromagnetic object is inside the magnet, no further pulling force is experienced. The boomerang effect reported in some accidents is based on the fact that the object is accelerating, gaining speed while approaching the isocenter, and will pass the

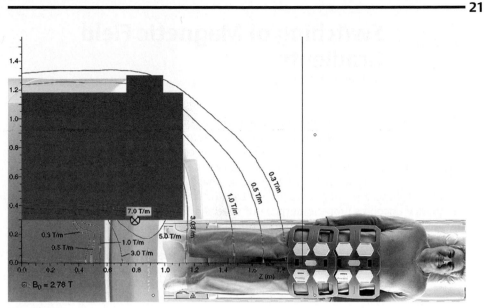

Figure 9-1

same if there is no counterforce stopping the motion. The object then continues to fly through the magnet until its kinetic energy is compensated by the potential energy of the force pulling the object back into the center of the magnet. At that point, the object will change directions and fly back toward the isocenter of the magnet. **Figure 9-2** presents another recent example of the all too common case of the nightshift attempting to polish the floor of the magnet room, unsupervised.

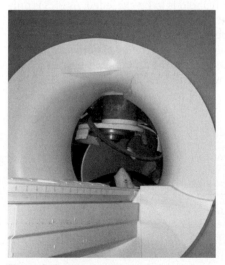

Figure 9-2

10 Switching of Magnetic Field Gradients

Wolfgang R. Nitz

There are several occasions in MR imaging where, although for a very short time period, a variation in the magnetic field strength is required within the imaging volume, either to have different Larmor frequencies to selectively excite the protons (the spin of the nucleus of the hydrogen atoms bound to water or fat) of a given slice, or to have different Larmor frequencies to prepare a phase shift for the purpose of spatial encoding (phase encoding) or different Larmor frequencies during data acquisition (frequency encoding) for the purpose of spatial encoding. Although the strength of the magnetic field gradient is given by the desired frequency bandwidth during excitation or spatial encoding, the faster the final gradient amplitude can be achieved, the shorter the echo time. This results in a shortening of the echo train, increasing SNR and thus improving image quality.

♦ Stimulation

A change in magnetic field over time is termed dB/dt. According to Maxwell's law, this dB/dt will induce a current in a conductive loop. Because the patient represents multiple potential although weak conductive loops, at a certain dB/dt value [either large change in amplitude (dB) and/or in a very short time (dt)], the induced current might be large enough to stimulate peripheral nerves. Because dB/dt values can be calculated prior to sequence execution, a software monitor compares the calculated value with the peripheral nerve stimulation (PNS) threshold and prohibits the execution of a pulse sequence or will issue a warning if the threshold is to be exceeded. As PNS is only a function of dB/dt, there is no dependence on the overall magnetic field strength.

Figure 10–1 illustrates the local change in magnetic field during spatial encoding in the coronal direction. In this example, the field is higher toward the head of the patient and lower as compared with B_0 toward the feet of the patient. The difference is termed dB. The change in the magnetic field over time is the above-mentioned dB/dt, which is responsible for inducing a current in the patient's body that may lead to PNS.

♦ Acoustic Noise

The law describing the mechanical force on a wire carrying a current through a magnetic field is called the Lorentz force. For example, for a magnetic field gradient along the direction of

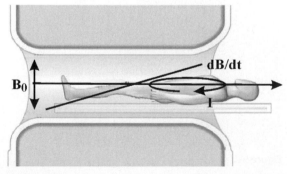

Figure 10–1

the main field (z-direction), the Lorentz force will cause one end of the gradient coil to be compressed and the other end to be expanded. Although made out of solid material, the gradient coil will vibrate due to the fast switching of currents (creating magnetic field gradients), causing the noise heard during an MR exam. As the Lorentz force is proportional to the current through the wire and the strength of the main magnetic field, one would expect the generated acoustic noise at higher field strength to be stronger if no counteracting measures are performed (e.g., additional damping or any action to keep the vibrating gradient coil from generating air-pressure waves).

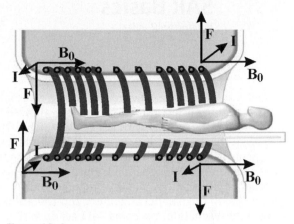

Figure 10–2

Figure 10–2 illustrates the simple case of a local change in magnetic field in the caudocranial direction achieved by sending a current (I) through a gradient coil. Increasing the field toward the head and decreasing the field toward the patient's feet is achieved by changing the direction of the gradient coil windings causing the current flow counterclockwise caudally and clockwise cranially. The direction of the main field is indicated by B_0, and according to Lorentz, the mechanical force (F) of the flowing current (I) interacting with the main magnetic field (B_0) will try to compress the gradient coil at the location of the patient's feet and will try to expand the gradient coil at the location of the patient's head. Although the mechanical force is counteracted by several measures, a small vibration remains, causing the creation of a sound wave every time a current is sent to any of the various gradient windings.

11 SAR Basics

Wolfgang R. Nitz

When fat and water are exposed to a strong external magnetic field, the spins of the hydrogen atom nuclei (a single proton) are allowed to take two positions. They may align themselves parallel with the field, which is the low-energy position, or they may align themselves antiparallel with the field, which is the less desired higher-energy position. The difference in population, as more spins will be aligned parallel as compared with antiparallel, represents the longitudinal magnetization. To get a signal, an RF excitation pulse is required that provides exactly the energy difference between the parallel alignment and the antiparallel alignment of the nuclear spins. After excitation, the spins fall back into their original position, emitting the energy as an MR signal. The RF pulse will also interact with water molecules. Because the weak molecular dipole moments of water try to align to the flux lines of the applied RF field, their rotational motion is accelerated. An increase in motion is equivalent to an increase in kinetic energy and represents an increase in temperature. This is comparable with the energy required to put a book on a higher shelf. In doing so, the book is getting a higher potential energy, which is the product of height and weight. However, we need more energy as we have to erect our own body and lift the weight of our arm in addition to putting energy into the book (and it is going to warm us up).

The power that is absorbed by the patient during MR imaging is characterized by the specific absorption rate (SAR). The order of magnitude of the power deposition during MR imaging is close to the human metabolic rate. An average-size person requires ~8000 kJ per day to exist in a resting state. This translates into a continuous power all day long of ~90 W. This power is known as the basal metabolic rate. The international guideline (IEC 60601–2-33) on safety requirements in MR assumes 2 W/kg whole-body SAR exposure as being no burden to the patient (normal mode), which is 160 W for a patient weight of 176 lb for the duration of a scan.

The classical perspective of the SAR mechanism considers the interaction of the electrical component and the magnetic component of the RF field with the biological tissue of the patient's body. Various conductive pathways along soft tissue allow resistive losses, and multiple water molecules are craving for some guidance by rapidly changing RF flux lines. The likelihood of interaction, represented by the SAR value, scales with the fifth power of the patient's circumference. That is bad news for the obese patient. Physical restraint using a nonconductive corset would help but is of course impractical. The likelihood of interaction, represented by the SAR value, also scales with the conductivity inside the patient. Because body fat has little electrical conductivity as compared with body fluid, that is good news for the obese patient. Unfortunately, the effect of conductivity on SAR is only linear as compared with the fifth power of the patient's circumference. Dehydration would help but is of course also impractical.

For T1-weighted brain studies at 3 T, one practical solution to reduce SAR is to replace spin-echo (SE) imaging with gradient-echo (GRE) imaging **(Fig. 11–1)**. Using a

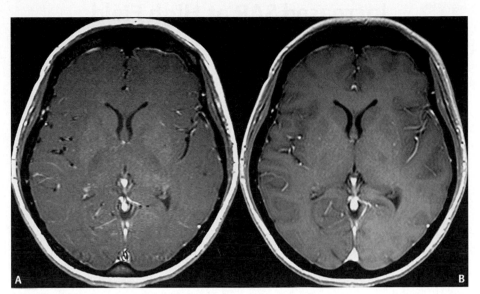

Figure 11–1

single 70-degree excitation pulse every 255 msec **(Fig. 11–1B)** as compared with a 90- to 180-degree combination every 330 msec **(Fig. 11–1A)** will reduce the SAR by almost 85%. As an additional benefit, the gray/white matter contrast is improved as well at 3 T when selecting a GRE as compared with an SE protocol.

12 Increased SAR at High Field
Wolfgang R. Nitz

To flip the spin of a proton (hydrogen atom nucleus) to the less preferred antiparallel position, the RF coil has to provide the energy difference between these two positions, which is characterized by the frequency of the RF pulse. The SAR for a patient is proportional to the square of that frequency. As compared with a 1.5 T system, potential SAR thus increases by a factor of four for a 3 T system. Using the example of stacking a bookshelf, the shelf will now be so high that you may have to step up a ladder to put the book on the higher shelf. This would be substantially more exercise than if you just had to raise your arm to put the book on the shelf. With regard to the patient, there is no reason to be concerned. The safety requirements are still the same whether it is a 1.5 T system or a 3 T system. The patient will not be exposed to an SAR beyond the safety requirements. However, measures will have to be taken, as discussed later, that compensate for the potential increase due to the higher resonance frequency. For example, the same exact scan often cannot be run at both 1.5 and 3 T, simply because of SAR limitations. A scan that has high SAR at 1.5 T cannot be employed without changes at 3 T, as SAR limits would be exceeded.

At a certain point, it is very inconvenient to explain and hard to depict excitation, refocusing, and flipping of spins on a quantum mechanical level. It is valid to consider the difference between parallel-aligned and antiparallel-aligned spins forming one (net) longitudinal magnetization. That longitudinal magnetization behaves like a rotating magnetic gyroscope that starts precessing as soon as it is flipped away from the longitudinal direction. It is no surprise that in calculating the precessional frequency of that longitudinal magnetization, it matches the Larmor frequency of the quantum mechanical model. It is the magnetic component of the RF that will flip the longitudinal magnetization if the frequency of the RF is matching the Larmor frequency within the tissue. Flipping the longitudinal magnetization perpendicular to the main field direction is termed a *90-degree pulse*, and the longitudinal magnetization will then become the transverse magnetization. The latter will continue to precess with the Larmor frequency and will induce an MR signal as long as the T2-relaxation time will permit. The magnetic field component of the RF that does the flipping is called B_1. The SAR is proportional to the square of the amplitude of that B_1 field.

In summary, SAR is proportional to

- the power of two for the system's resonance frequency.
- the power of two for the B_1 amplitude of the RF field.
- the power of five for the patient's circumference.
- the patient's average conductivity.

One potential measure to reduce the SAR is to decrease the B_1 amplitude of the RF field by using low excitation angles or refocusing angles below 180 degrees. **Figure 12–1** demonstrates the loss in contrast as a consequence of using low-angle refocusing pulses for a patient with multiple simple renal and hepatic cysts: **(A)** is

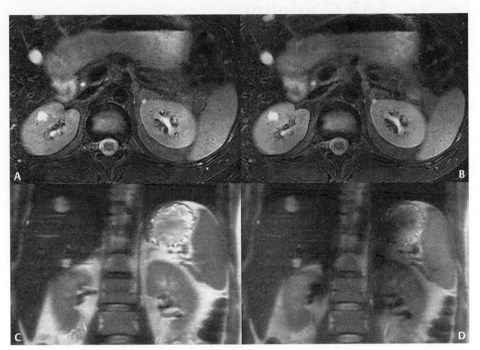

Figure 12–1

an axial FSE acquisition using a 180-degree refocusing angle, whereas (**B**) was acquired using a 137-degree refocusing angle; (**C**) presents a coronal half-Fourier acquisition single-shot turbo-spin echo (HASTE) image in the same patient using a 180-degree refocusing angle, and (**D**) demonstrates the contrast for the same slice and identical technique except for the use of a refocusing angle of only 90 degrees. The changes in this instance due to a reduction in refocusing angle are much more evident in the HASTE image comparison.

13 SAR Guidelines

Wolfgang R. Nitz

The international standard [IEC 60601–2-33 (September 9, 2001)] on "particular requirements for the safety of magnetic resonance equipment for medical diagnosis" considers SAR threshold values for three different modes: the normal mode, the first level, and the "forbidden" second level. Exposure below the normal-mode SAR level is assumed to cause no physiologic stress to the patient. For SAR values within the range of the first level, medical supervision of the patient is required. Specifically, the system has to indicate that it has to switch into first level to execute the requested protocol, and the operator must acknowledge the note in order for the system to continue.

Normal mode:

- Up to 2 W/kg whole-body exposure
- Up to 2 to 10 W/kg partial body exposure, depending on the ratio between exposed and unexposed patient mass
- Up to 3.2 W/kg for head exposure
- Up to 10 W/kg for local SAR within the head/trunk region
- Up to 20 W/kg for local SAR values within the extremities

Body core temperature is not to increase beyond 0.5°C.

First-level mode:

- Up to 4 W/kg whole-body exposure
- Up to 4 to 10 W/kg partial body exposure, depending on the ratio between exposed and unexposed patient mass
- Up to 3.2 W/kg for head exposure
- Up to 10 W/kg for local SAR within the head/trunk region
- Up to 20 W/kg for local SAR values within the extremities

Body core temperature is not to increase beyond 1°C.

Values are averaged over a 6-min time frame. For a period of 10 sec, the averaged SAR may exceed up to 3 times the level of the current mode. These levels are valid for a bore temperature of up to 77°F and decrease linearly to 0 for the normal mode and 2 W/kg for the first level for a bore temperature of 91.4°F.

The software on the MR system will calculate and compare all possible limits for the selected mode and will in general indicate the most critical value. If the critical value exceeds the level of the selected mode, suggestions are made to the operator regarding which scan parameters to change (and to what value) to stay within the guidelines. No MR system will allow the execution of a protocol that exceeds the guidelines of the country where the scanner is located.

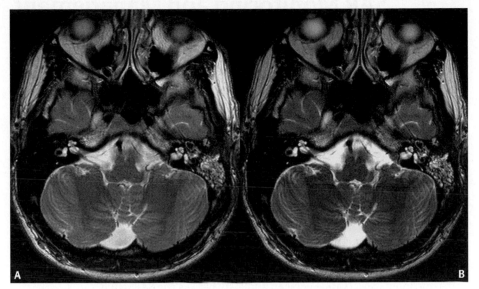

Figure 13–1

The T2-weighted FSE study displayed in **Fig. 13–1** reveals opacification by fluid of the mastoid air cells and middle ear cavity on the left. This case provides one example of how to optimize image quality for the same measurement time and the same SAR level. **Figure 13–1A** has been acquired with a 4.21-sec repetition time and an echo train length of 11 for a scan time of 4:01 min. The effective echo time was 73 msec. **Figure 13–1B** has been acquired with a 4-sec repetition time and an echo train length of 19. To have the same number of slices (19), two scan concatenations were used (two separate scans were acquired) leading to a measurement time of 2 × 2:12 min. The improvement in contrast is due to the longer effective echo time of this study, 104 msec, as compared with the TE of 73 msec of the comparative study. The improvement in SNR is likely due to the slightly extended measurement time of 4:24 min. As a general rule, SNR is an almost linear function of spatial resolution and measurement time for a given field strength.

14 SAR Monitoring and Management
Wolfgang R. Nitz

SAR is primarily a function of field strength, amplitude of the RF pulse, patient conductivity, patient circumference, and, finally, the patient's effective region within the RF field (transmitter coil design). The latter considers the patient position relative to the transmitter coil. As a safety precaution, vendors perform mathematical simulations using various human models to verify compliance with the safety guidelines. The various limits are checked prior to execution of the sequence. The user will have guided choices to start the measurement. All vendors must have at least a dual path to verify that the SAR limits are not exceeded. The first path consists of a direct measurement. The energy lost within the system is estimated during the adjustment. Based on these values, the energy absorbed by the patient is calculated. The second path will take the transmitter adjustment values, the results of the simulations, and the patient's weight, age, height, and position to come up with an estimation of the energy likely to be absorbed by the patient. Whatever value is delivered by any of these paths, the most conservative is taken and displayed as the SAR value.

Any RF pulse within the protocol to be executed will contribute to the SAR. This can be spatial saturation pulses, fat saturation pulses, inversion pulses, magnetization transfer saturation pulses, excitation, or refocusing pulses.

In cases where the SAR limit exceeds the guidelines, the following measures will help:

- Prolong the TR (prolonging the measurement time), which will help to spread the energy over a longer time window.

- Reduce the number of slices, which will reduce the number of RF pulses for the same measurement time.

- Reduce the refocusing flip angle, which will decrease the B_1 field amplitude. This factor is contributing with a power of two to the SAR value.

- Reduce the echo train length (ETL, or turbo factor), which will lead to fewer RF pulses for the same TR, spreading the delivered energy over a longer time window (at the expense of increasing measurement time).

- Use low SAR pulses. The B_1 amplitude will dictate the speed of flipping. A short RF pulse with large B_1 field amplitude will have the same flipping or refocusing effect as a long RF pulse with smaller B_1 field amplitude. Because B_1 is contributing by the power of two to the SAR, a reduction in amplitude causes a significant reduction in the SAR value. On the other hand, longer RF pulses will lead to prolonged echo times, which prolong the length of echo trains, resulting in reduced signal. The latter is due to T2 decay. Longer echo trains or longer echo times will also lead to a higher sensitivity to flow, motion, and susceptibility artifacts.

- Place a pause before or after the measurement. Some vendors provide the option to select in advance a pause at the end of the measurement. That pause will be considered in the SAR calculation, averaged over time, and may result in the scan being within SAR guidelines. The same is applicable for an alternative delay prior

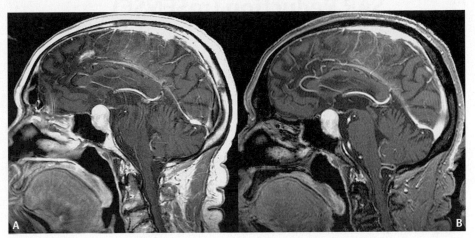

Figure 14–1

to executing multiple measurements in conjunction with contrast enhancement. Some vendors offer an SAR look-ahead to avoid any enforced pausing between measurements.

Another alternative to reduce the SAR is to omit the RF refocusing pulse and use GRE imaging instead of SE imaging. **Figure 14–1** presents postcontrast scans from a patient with a macroadenoma: **(A)** was acquired in 3:23 min using a spin-echo acquisition scheme providing a spatial resolution of $0.7 \times 0.8 \times 3$ mm^3; the measurement time for **(B)** was 1:32 min using a gradient echo acquisition scheme (with markedly lower SAR) providing a spatial resolution of $0.8 \times 0.8 \times 2$ mm^3.

15 SAR Reduction (mSENSE)
Wolfgang R. Nitz

Energy per unit time is called power. The power absorbed within the patient's body will cause an increase in body or local tissue temperature. This power divided by the patient's body weight is called the specific absorption rate (SAR). Staying within SAR guidelines is the major criteria for sequence and protocol selection in high-field imaging (3 T). The energy of each saturation pulse, inversion pulse, excitation pulse, and refocusing pulse for each Fourier line to be measured will increase the energy of molecular motion within the body, as characterized by the body temperature. This will finally lead to a response of the human temperature regulatory system. It has been verified that if the energy per unit time is delivered slow enough, the regulatory system will have no problem coping with that additional energy.

There are several measures that can be used to reduce the SAR value. One potential way is to use parallel imaging. This approach will only help if the parallel imaging is not used to reduce measurement time but solely used to reduce the SAR value (by adjusting the measurement time to remain constant)!

Parallel imaging is defined as using the spatial distribution of surface coils or imaging matrix elements in the direction of phase encoding. This eliminates certain phase-encoding steps that are otherwise required to retrieve spatial information. The method is called *parallel imaging*, or PAT, as each coil is measuring the signal from the patient's body simultaneously and in parallel to one another.

As an example, the measurement of every second Fourier line is skipped if an acceleration factor of two is selected. That acceleration factor is also called a "PAT" factor in this context. This measure corresponds with a selection of a 50% FOV in the direction of phase encoding. If the object to be imaged extends beyond that FOV, foldover artifacts will be the consequence. However, these artifacts will be eliminated using a PAT image reconstruction algorithm.

The image-based PAT algorithm is called *SENSE* (sensitivity encoding). Hidden from the user, each coil is "parallel to other coils," sampling the signal and reconstructing an image with all the foldover artifacts (e.g., for two coils: image no. 1, image no. 2). The signal received by each coil will vary depending on the sensitivity profile of the coil. The foldover artifacts will also depend on coil position. Because each of the coil elements has a different spatial position, the foldover artifacts will look different for each of the images constructed. That appearance will allow a differentiation between true signal and foldover artifacts.

The following represents a simple set of two equations used to calculate the true signal and to reconstruct an image without foldover artifacts. For example, for two coils, measured image no. 1 = (true signal + foldover artifacts) × sensitivity profile no. 1, and measured image no. 2 = (true signal + foldover artifacts) × sensitivity profile no. 2.

Skipping the measurement of Fourier lines will also cause a loss in SNR, as each measurement contains information about the entire slice. Each Fourier line can be considered an additional acquisition. The loss in SNR using "parallel imaging" has been a major limitation in the past for PAT applications. This is overcome using the increase in SNR when going to higher field strength (3 T). If SAR becomes an issue, PAT applications can be helpful in reducing the number of RF pulses while keeping the measurement time constant.

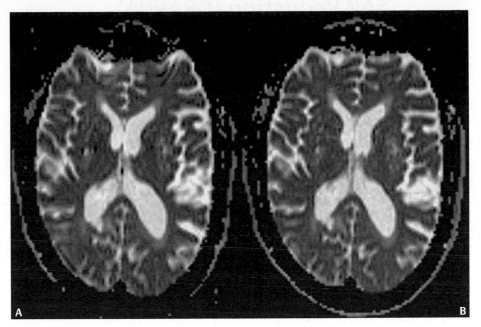

Figure 15–1

In **Fig. 15–1**, T2-weighted echo planar images are shown from the exam of a patient with multiple strokes. In this case, mSENSE (**Fig. 15–1B**, with no PAT applied in **Fig. 15–1A**) does not lead to a reduction in SAR, as no additional RF is applied to generate another gradient echo, but the ETL is reduced, leading to a reduction of the susceptibility artifacts. Note the reduced spatial distortion anteriorly in the image with PAT.

16 SAR Reduction (GRAPPA)

Wolfgang R. Nitz

Parallel imaging (PAT) is the use of the different positions of surface coil elements to retrieve spatial information that otherwise would have been measured with additional phase-encoding steps. Skipping the measurement of Fourier lines corresponds with a reduction in the FOV in the direction of phase encoding, as previously noted. The image-based PAT algorithm SENSE compares the images provided by each coil element to identify and eliminate the foldover artifacts. It is also possible to eliminate these artifacts prior to Fourier transformation. These PAT algorithms are called k-space–based parallel imaging reconstruction techniques (with one example being GRAPPA). In conventional Cartesian-type sampled k-space, each Fourier line represents the information for a specific spatial frequency. That is, the center Fourier line contains information about the overall signal from the slice and the distribution in the direction of frequency encoding. The first and the last Fourier lines contain the information about the highest spatial frequency in the direction of phase encoding as selected by the user. The Fourier lines between outer k-space and the center of k-space contain the information of various spatial frequencies, from coarse structures to smaller details, which are necessary to achieve an unambiguous signal assignment of higher spatial frequencies. As previously discussed, a linear combination of distributed coil elements in the direction of phase encoding can be used to reconstruct missing k-space lines.

Parallel imaging, either mSENSE or GRAPPA, can be used:

♦ to shorten measurement time (by reducing the number of Fourier lines to be measured), at the expense of SNR.

♦ to increase spatial resolution for the same measurement time. Be aware that in addition to the SNR loss correlated with the use of PAT, there is additional SNR loss due to smaller voxel size.

♦ to decrease SAR keeping the measurement time constant. This means to extend TR to keep the measurement time constant or to reduce the echo train length in FSE imaging.

♦ to decrease susceptibility artifacts in echo planar imaging (EPI) by reducing the echo train length while maintaining the measurement time.

Figure 16–1 demonstrates the case of a patient with a neoplasm involving the cerebellum. Illustrated is the path for image reconstruction. Parallel imaging (when a PAT factor of two is employed) is simply the use of a rectangular field of view, correlated with the skipping of Fourier lines. Employed in this manner, parallel imaging saves measurement time or, in cases where the measurement time is kept constant, reduces the SAR. Each Fourier line represents a spatial frequency.

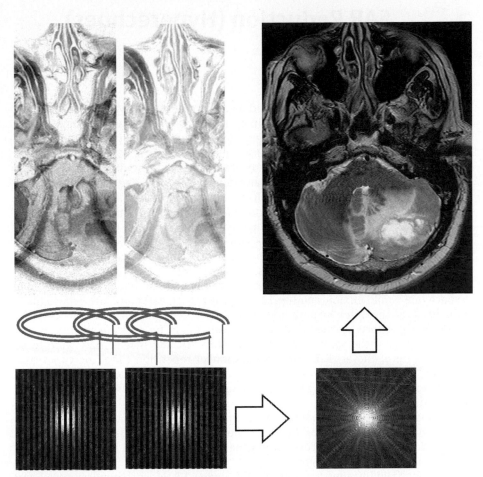

Figure 16–1

Coil elements distributed in the direction of phase encoding can be combined to retrieve spatial frequencies. The combined signals of these distributed coil elements can be used to reconstruct missing Fourier lines, and the Fourier transformation of the final k-space will, in most cases, lead to images without foldover artifacts.

17 SAR Reduction (Hyperechoes)
Wolfgang R. Nitz

In viewing T2-weighted images, it should be noted that starting with an echo time of 60 msec and moving up to an echo time of 120 msec will gradually increase the T2 weighting. The basic contrast remains unchanged: cerebrospinal fluid (CSF) is hyperintense, white matter is hypointense, and gray matter is not as hypointense as white matter. This observation triggered the invention of using multiple phase-encoded echoes to fill multiple k-space lines after a single excitation. The slight variations in signal due to T2 decay and the slight different weighting of k-space lines were considered negligible. That invention was termed *RARE* (rapid acquisition with relaxation enhancement). With improvements in hardware, this technique was reinvented and implemented by major vendors as TSE (turbo spin-echo) or FSE (fast spin-echo). Fast spin-echo imaging has replaced conventional spin-echo imaging for all proton density- and T2-weighted applications.

Early scientific reports cautioned against the use of FSE imaging because each k-space line would exhibit another T2 weighting, with early and late echoes likely to be used for the outer k-space lines containing the high spatial frequencies, the details. Early reports warned that small objects might be overlooked. This would have been true if the same imaging parameters, TR and matrix size, were to be applied. State-of-the-art FSE imaging uses longer repetition time (increased contrast) and increased matrix size (better spatial resolution). This outweighs the consequences of T2 decay during k-space filling, leading to an even higher sensitivity in depicting small lesions.

SNR and CNR are mainly determined in the center of k-space. Placing the shorter echoes and the later echoes of the multiecho train in the outer lines of k-space will have no consequences if the contrast in general is improved and if the global spatial resolution is selected to be higher.

With high-field imaging, the multiple 180-degree RF refocusing pulses pose a real challenge with respect to the SAR. A common solution is the use of low refocusing flip angles, which lead to a considerable reduction in SAR at the cost of the SNR.

With the idea of concentrating on the center of k-space, techniques have surfaced that allow the "important" signals encoding for the center of k-space to be fully refocused. This avoids SNR loss, while echoes at the beginning and toward the end of the echo train, which encode the more peripheral parts of k-space, are generated using low flip angle refocusing pulses. The sequence acronyms for these techniques are variable flip angle TSE, hyperechoes, TRAPS (transitions between pseudo steady states), and SPACE (sampling perfection with application optimized contrast by using different flip angle evolutions).

The application of multiple refocusing pulses with small flip angles will in general lead to a more and more complex constructive superimposition of multiple refocusing pathways. It has been published that, as a surprising consequence, variable flip angle refocusing FSE may achieve a higher signal intensity for the center of k-space as compared with a fully refocused FSE sequence. Because the resulting signal can be regarded as an echo of echoes, the term *hyperecho* has been introduced.

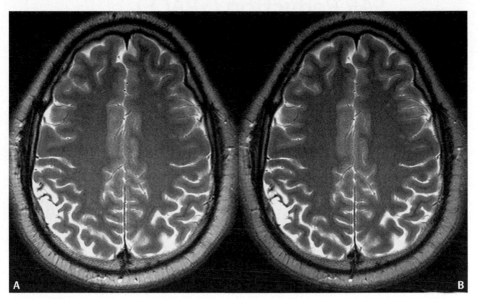

Figure 17–1

The use of parallel imaging and SAR reduction with hyperechoes is demonstrated in **Fig. 17–1**. Both images represent a spatial resolution of $0.45 \times 0.64 \times 3$ mm^3 and were acquired within 79 sec: image **(A)** represents one slice out of 18 using 89% of the allowed SAR limit; image **(B)** has been acquired using hyperechoes and allowed a package of 36 slices using 66% of the allowed SAR limit. This is an impressive example of the use of hyperechoes to reduce the SAR.

18 SAR Reduction (SPACE)
Wolfgang R. Nitz

The majority of MR techniques, especially for brain imaging, are based on SE imaging methods. This is mainly due to the resistance of the SE technique to image artifacts from anatomy-related static-field inhomogeneities and the ability to achieve true T2 weighting. A theoretically possible major benefit of clinical MR brain imaging would be a true volume acquisition with the potential of retrospectively reconstructing high-spatial resolution images in any arbitrary orientation. In conjunction with conventional SE imaging, such an approach would lead to impractical measurement times. With the introduction of FSE techniques, the three-dimensional approach became feasible, but the power deposition is relatively high and will likely be prohibitive for imaging at higher field strengths such as 3 T. Reducing the flip angle of the refocusing RF pulse in an FSE sequence acquisition scheme has been demonstrated as a means of addressing high RF power deposition at the cost of SNR. However, signal levels tend to oscillate from echo to echo, potentially leading to image artifacts. It has been demonstrated that continuously varying the flip angle of the refocusing RF pulses, individually adjusted, can dampen or eliminate the signal oscillations thus reducing imaging artifacts. Small flip angle refocusing will produce a signal composition of multiple echo paths, the previously mentioned hyperechoes. It has also been demonstrated that the SE amplitude approaches a temporary steady state that then slowly decays due to relaxation. Because the "steady state" is actually only temporary, it is referred to as a pseudo steady state. The approach of using a train of variable refocusing flip angles in an arrangement such that the echoes close to the center of k-space are fully refocused is called *TRAPS* (transitions between pseudo steady states). Using a flip angle series that yields a constant signal for the majority of the spatially encoding echo train, taking into account the relaxation during data sampling, will further improve image quality. This optimization requires knowledge of the relaxation values for the tissue to be imaged. Application-specific flip angle evolution, maintaining the desired contrast even in ultralong echo trains in combination with a 3D FSE imaging acquisition scheme, has been named *SPACE* (sampling perfection with application optimized contrasts using different flip angle evolutions). This method provides for the necessary reduction in SAR, taking advantage of a volume acquisition and optimizing the achievable CNR for a specific application.

Figure 18-1, which was acquired using the SPACE technique [3D FSE imaging using continuously varying flip angles for the refocusing RF pulses, adapted for the specific application

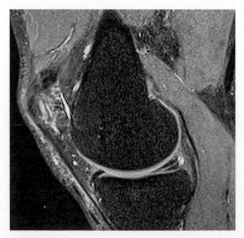

Figure 18-1

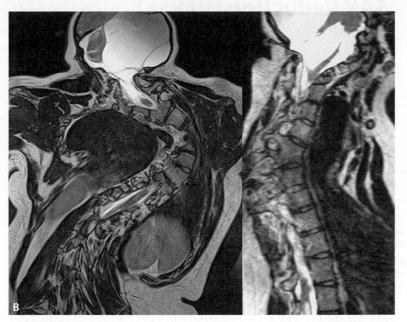

Figure 18–2

(considering relaxation effects)] and a spatial resolution of $0.6 \times 0.6 \times 0.6$ mm^3, well depicts a meniscal tear.

An additional impressive application of the volume acquisition using a fast 3D SE scheme like SPACE is shown in **Fig. 18–2**. The achievable isotropic resolution of the original volume acquisition [one partition shown in **(A)**] allows for the retrospective reconstruction of a plane along the course of this tortuous spine **(B)**.

19 SAR Reduction (VERSE)

Wolfgang R. Nitz

A 90-degree RF excitation pulse "flips" the longitudinal magnetization into the transverse plane. The transverse magnetization will rotate with the Larmor frequency and will dephase as a consequence of spin-spin interaction (T2) and local magnetic field inhomogeneities. The effect due to local field inhomogeneities is likely stable in time and fixed in location and can be rephased using a 180-degree RF pulse. To excite and rephase, energy is transferred into the patient, and the energy per unit time that remains within the patient is called the specific absorption rate (SAR). While imaging at 3 T can theoretically provide a twofold improvement in SNR compared with 1.5 T, it is also burdened by a fourfold increase in RF power. The amplitude of the RF pulse contributes to the SAR by the power of two. A large RF amplitude provides a specified flip angle or rephasing within a short RF duration, whereas a low RF amplitude requires a longer duration of the RF pulse to achieve the same effect. Common approaches to reducing RF power include using a lower flip angle for the rephasing RF pulses or prolonging the RF duration. Reducing the refocusing flip angle produces signals from stimulated echo pathways that have mixed T1 and T2 contrast as well as lower overall signal levels, thus usually leading to a loss in CNR. Stretching RF pulses results in longer echo spacing and thus exacerbates the effects of relaxation through the echo train.

Most of the RF pulses have their maximum halfway through the duration of the pulse. Any measure during that time leading to a reduction in RF amplitude will significantly reduce the SAR. **Figure 19–1A** illustrates the course of a "normal" RF pulse in comparison with **Fig. 19–1B**, where a "low SAR" RF pulse is used. The basic idea is to use a "short" RF duration at the beginning and at the end of the RF pulse and a "long" RF duration at the time of the expected peak of the RF pulse **(Fig. 19–1C)**. This will reduce the RF amplitude at a point in time where the SAR contribution is usually

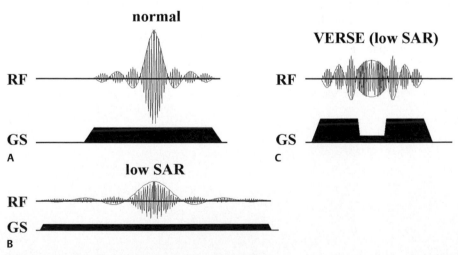

Figure 19–1 RF, radio frequency; GS, slice select gradient.

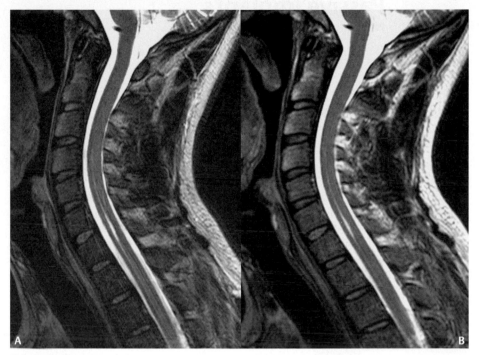

Figure 19–2

significant. This concept has been named variable-rate selective excitation (VERSE). In **Fig. 19–2**, sagittal images of the cervical spine are presented in a patient with hydromyelia. These were acquired using FSE technique with a repetition time of 3.5 sec, an echo time of 123 msec, and a spatial resolution of $0.38 \times 0.5 \times 3$ mm^3, for a scan time of $2 \times 1{:}49$ min: **(A)** was acquired using prolonged "low SAR" RF pulses, where-as **(B)** was acquired using the VERSE scheme. There are several observations comparing these two acquisitions. The VERSE scheme uses shorter RF refocusing pulses leading to shorter echo spacing. This will lead to acquisition of more echoes at shorter echo times leading to an overall improvement in SNR. The smoothed appearances of some small structures indicate that the slice profile of the VERSE scheme might be slightly affected, leading to increased partial volume effects.

20 Passive Implants
Wolfgang R. Nitz

Considering the safety of passive implants, three primary interactions with the MR system have to be discussed:

- static magnetic field
- gradient field
- RF field

Implants classified as "non-ferromagnetic" are deemed safe. As an example, the spinal rods shown in **Fig. 20–1** (courtesy of Peter Brehm, Herzogenaurach, Germany) are made of non-ferromagnetic alloy and will not interact with the static magnetic field. The same is valid for the artificial hip prosthesis shown in **Fig. 20–2**. In most cases, these types of implants present no hazard to the patient. Implants are characterized as being MR safe using ex vivo testing as described by the American Society for Testing

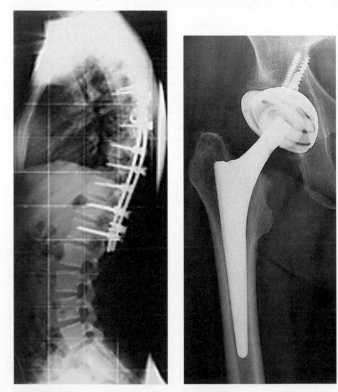

Figure 20–1   Figure 20–2

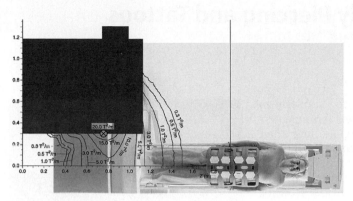

Figure 20–3

and Materials (ASTM). In the case of ferromagnetism, two interactions with the static magnetic field have to be considered:

♦ torque, which is a function of the field strength

♦ translational attraction, which is a function of the fringe field distribution

Brain aneurysm clips represent a classic contraindication for MR imaging due to at least one reported fatality where a ferromagnetic aneurysm clip tore a middle cerebral artery. Recent publications have documented that at least those aneurysm clips made from titanium alloys can be considered MR safe. As outlined in Case 9, the torque on a ferromagnetic object inside a 3 T magnet increases by a factor of four as compared with a 1.5 T system. The translational attractive force on a ferromagnetic object is a function of the product of the local magnetic field strength and the magnetic gradient field, as shown in **Fig. 20–3**. The translational force approximately triples on a 3 T system as compared with a 1.5 T system. Orthodontic appliances pose a potential risk during MR imaging because of forces on metallic objects within the static magnetic field. Steel ligature wires and arch wires made of cobalt chromium, titanium molybdenum, nickel-titanium, and brass alloys have shown no or negligible forces within the magnetic field. Steel retainer wire bonds should be checked to ensure secure attachment prior to an MR imaging exam as translational forces are estimated to be 27 to 75 times as high as gravitational forces on these objects.

The switching of magnetic field gradients potentially causing peripheral nerve stimulation is of less concern for conductive implants. Heating of implants and similar devices may occur if they are made from conductive materials and have an elongated shape or are arranged in loops.

It is the coupling with the RF used for saturation, excitation, and refocusing that may cause tissue heating in the vicinity of the implant or even heating of the implant itself. The heating is a function of the local SAR value and of the geometric arrangement with respect to the RF transmitting coil.

Recent reports indicate that aneurysm coils for example may cause a noticeable heating of their environment. Conductive shapes of the dimension of half the wavelength are considered a potential hazard as they may resonate with the RF field. The RF wavelength in water is ~52 cm for a 1.5 T system. For a 3 T system, that wavelength is only 26 cm. Conductive structures as short as 13 cm may resonate with the RF field, causing currents within conductive implants that have the potential to heat the implant itself.

21 Body Piercing and Tattoos
Wolfgang R. Nitz

Piercings can be treated similarly to passive implants. Their ferromagnetism is usually negligible, and their size is usually too small to interact with the switching of the magnetic field gradients or with the RF field. They will cause significant artifacts, but they do not present a potential hazard to the patients. There are no reports of body piercings being torn and pulled into the magnet, and there

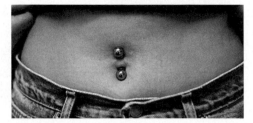

Figure 21–1

are no reports of these piercings becoming hot. Because these piercings are partially outside of biological tissue, the shorter wavelength of a 3 T system should be of no concern (**Fig. 21–1**).

The discussion on tattoos (**Fig. 21–2**) and permanent cosmetics is somewhat controversial. Problems related to MR procedures and tattoos are reported to be associated with the use of iron oxide or other metal-based pigments. A few cases are published where patients with tattoos who underwent MR procedures experienced transient skin irritation, cutaneous swelling, or heating sensations. There are studies reporting that ~1.5% of patients with permanent cosmetics will experience problems associated with MR imaging.

It has also been reported that decorative tattoos tend to cause more severe problems, including first- and second-degree burns. Due to the relatively remote possibility of an incident occurring in a patient with permanent cosmetics or a tattoo and to the relatively minor short-term complications reported so far, the patient should be informed about a possible reaction but then permitted to undergo MR imaging. The application of ice packs or a wet towel to the site of the tattoo has been suggested to reduce the possibility of thermal injury, although there are no empirical data to date to support this recommendation.

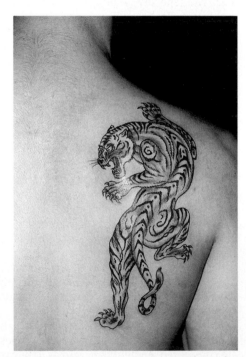

Figure 21–2

22 Active Implants
Wolfgang R. Nitz

Cardiac pacemakers are the most common electronically activated implants found in patients. **Figures 22–1** and **22–2** present x-ray images of two possible arrangements. Similar to passive implants, with regard to possible interactions with the MR system, the static magnetic field, the fringe field, and the RF field must be considered.

Any ferromagnetic components within the pulse generator may result in a movement of the object. Reed switch function is usually unpredictable and may result in ventricular fibrillation, rapid pacing, asynchronous pacing,

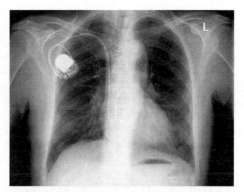

Figure 22–1

inhibition of pacing output, alteration of programming, or possible damage to the pacemaker circuitry. Several studies on non-pacemaker-dependent patients indicate that certain pacemakers may be MR safe. However, all of these studies were based on empirical and not analytical experiments, thus conclusions based on the methods of analysis presented are problematic.

The lateral course of the lead may interact with the axial E-field component of the RF field. The craniocaudal extension of the lead will present no potential hazard as long as it is close to the isocenter of the magnet. If the latter is not the case, the lead may couple with horizontal E-field components found in the vicinity of the RF transmit coil. For non-pacemaker-dependent patients this will, as empirically evaluated and published, not lead to any consequences, although several reports indicate a necessary readjustment of the pacing threshold values. Although the reported results are encouraging, clinicians must be aware that manufacturers do not claim that their devices are currently MR safe or MR compatible. There are no cardiac devices that have yet achieved FDA clearance for MR compatibility.

Addressing the same issue, there are several publications dealing with the safety of patients with neurostimulators during an MR examination, with the claim that MR imaging can be performed safely even at 3 T. According to the warning letter issued by the FDA in May 2005, the FDA received several reports of serious

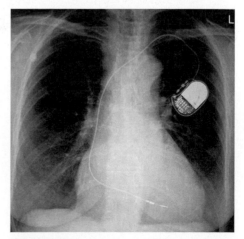

Figure 22–2

injury, including coma and permanent neurologic impairment, in patients with implanted neurologic stimulators who underwent an MR imaging procedure. The letter states that the mechanism for these adverse events is likely to involve heating of the surrounding tissue at the end of the lead wires, resulting in injury. Although these reports involved deep brain stimulators and vagus nerve stimulators, any type of implanted neurologic stimulator, such as spinal cord stimulators, peripheral nerve stimulators, and neuromuscular stimulators, could cause similar injuries.

With respect to imaging a patient with an active device using a 3 T MR system, the risk of an adverse event increases by several orders of magnitude compared with imaging at 1.5 T. The torque on any ferromagnetic object with an elongated shape will increase by a factor of four (see Case 9) as compared with a 1.5 T system. The translational force on any ferromagnetic material within the active implant will triple compared with 1.5 T when entering the bore of the magnet. Any RF coupling into pacing leads will deposit an amount of energy about four times higher on a 3 T system than on a 1.5 T system using identical RF pulses. Furthermore, the concern about a "dangerous" resonance is significantly increased because the critical half-wavelength within biological tissue is decreased from 26 cm for a 1.5 T system down to 13 cm on a 3 T system (see Case 20).

The majority of publications, generating the impression that MR imaging of patients with active implants may be safe, point out that their findings are highly specific to the MR system, the software version running the scanner, types of pacemakers and lead systems, and the geometrical arrangement of the device, the leads, and the patient within the RF resonator of the scanner. Furthermore, it is not valid to extrapolate the safety of devices evaluated at 1.5 T to a presumed safety profile at 3 T. Further studies will be required to verify the safety of those devices.

23 Intravascular and Intracavitary Implants

Wolfgang R. Nitz

Concerning the safety of interventional tools, the same criteria apply as for active or passive implants. Any ferromagnetic components within the interventional tool may result in a torque or translational movement. Any potential interaction with the RF field has to consider the higher frequency of the electromagnetic wave and the reduced wavelength.

There are a few interesting phenomena to be reported for MR-compatible puncture needles. A small susceptibility gradient due to the interventional tool is desired to create an artifact to allow for needle visibility during insertion. **Figure 23–1A** shows an image acquired with a GRE acquisition using an MR-compatible puncture needle (titanium alloy, DAUM Medical, Würzburg, Germany) on a 1.5 T system. The adjacent **Fig. 23–1B** has been acquired with a balanced GRE sequence (trueFISP, FIESTA, or bFFE) in a significantly shorter time (1.5 sec compared to 1 min). **Figures 23–1C** and **23–1D** have been acquired on a 3 T system using similar protocols. Comparing **(A)** and **(C)**, the gain in SNR when going to higher field strength (3 T) is obvious. Comparing **(B)** and **(D)**, the higher sensitivity to minor field inhomogeneities becomes evident, as destructive interference patterns are building up within the image acquired with a balanced GRE sequence on a 3 T system.

The risks associated with imaging a patient during an intervention on a 3 T MR system will increase compared with those associated with imaging at 1.5 T. The torque on any ferromagnetic object with an elongated shape will increase by a factor of four. The translational force on any ferromagnetic material within the interventional tool will triple.

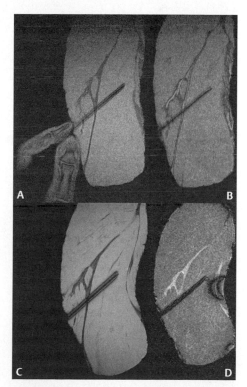

Figure 23–1

24 Brain: Spatial Resolution

Val M. Runge and Robert S. Case

3 T MR imaging represents one of the major forefronts of diagnostic neuroradiology today. However, information regarding routine clinical application is generally lacking due to rapid changes in instrumentation and the relatively small installed base. 3 T MR imaging offers higher SNR, which can be used either for improved spatial resolution or to scan faster, the latter being important for in-patient imaging. This has led to a divergence of protocols, with long, high-resolution scans on one end and

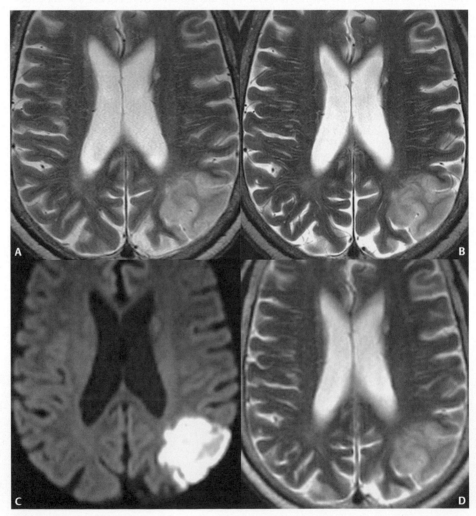

Figure 24–1

fast, lower-resolution scans on the other. A reduction in slice thickness for routine brain imaging is also an option with 3 T (with 2D multislice imaging), raising the question whether slice thickness will be reduced further in standard clinical practice (e.g., from 5 to 3 mm). Brain imaging at 3 T offers the potential for up to a factor of two improvement in signal SNR when compared with 1.5 T if a range of technical problems can be overcome. These include accentuated motion artifacts, SAR limits, and the prolongation of T1 with field strength.

Figure 24–1 presents MR images at 3 T of a 69-year-old woman with a past medical history of hypertension, tobacco abuse, and multiple previous transient ischemic attacks (TIAs). She presented to the emergency department with right-sided weakness for 2 days and difficulty with speech. The MR images demonstrate an early subacute infarct involving the posterior division of the left middle cerebral artery (MCA). **Figure 24–1A** illustrates the screening T2-weighted scan that we currently employ on the 3 T unit, using FSE technique with 3-mm sections through the entire brain in 72 sec. **Figure 24–1B** is from a second T2-weighted acquisition, with higher in-plane spatial resolution requiring a scan time of 2:39 (min:sec). Both scans employed a parallel imaging factor of two. **Figure 24–1C** is the diffusion-weighted scan, with the infarct demonstrating restricted diffusion (cytotoxic edema). **Figure 24–1D** presents one possible imaging approach for uncooperative patients. This T2-weighted scan employed a parallel-imaging factor of three, reduced in-plane resolution, and thicker slice section (5 mm) to achieve a scan time of 24 sec using FSE technique.

The improved SNR at 3 T leaves the neuroradiologist with a difficult decision, as illustrated in **Fig. 24–1**. High-resolution scans can be acquired with exquisite detail, or depending on the need and ability of the patient to cooperate, very rapid scan sequences can be acquired. Our current screening brain exam at 3 T includes a 2D 3-mm sagittal T1-weighted short TE gradient echo scan together with 3-mm axial FLAIR, T2-weighted, and diffusion-weighted scans requiring a total scan time just over 6 min. The FLAIR and T2-weighted scans are acquired with FSE technique. Using a lower-resolution approach, such as imaging with 5-mm slices, a further reduction in scan time is possible. The improved SNR at 3 T permits thinner sections to be acquired on a routine basis, combined with a reduction in scan time as compared with imaging at 1.5 T, decreasing motion artifacts as well as allowing improved imaging of uncooperative patients. This approach also allows rapid imaging when time is critical, such as in the diagnosis and management of acute stroke patients.

25 Brain: Slice Thickness

Val M. Runge and Robert S. Case

In this and many of the cases that follow, MR results at 1.5 and 3 T in the same patient will be directly compared, part of an institutional review board–approved study. The two MR units used in this comparison were located in adjacent clinical bays. Imaging at 1.5 T was performed on an 8-channel Magnetom Sonata system, with imaging at 3 T performed on an 8-channel Magnetom Trio system (Siemens Medical Solutions, Malvern, PA, USA). The gradient coils on these two MR units are identical. These are actively shielded, with a 40 mT/m gradient field strength and a slew rate of 200 T·m^{-1}·s^{-1}. The head coils used were of similar design, both 8-channel high-resolution head array coils (Invivo, Orlando, FL, USA). These two MR systems are as near identically matched as currently possible and represent the state of the art for 8-channel brain imaging at both field strengths.

Figure 25–1 illustrates the improved SNR at 3 T and its implications in regard to slice thickness. 3 T scans with varying slice thicknesses (5, 2.5, and 1 mm) are compared with imaging at 1.5 T with a 5-mm slice thickness. The images are from a 36-year-old poorly controlled diabetic with known atherosclerotic vascular disease. They show a 1.5-cm area of vasogenic edema consistent with an early subacute segmental anterior cerebral artery infarction (arrow, **Fig. 25–1C**). This area was positive (with marked abnormal high signal intensity) as well on the diffusion-weighted scan (not shown). In addition, there is a tiny remote cavitated left frontal white matter infarct. FSE heavily T2-weighted images are illustrated with TR, TE, bandwidth, and number of echoes held constant. Scan time was also held constant, with each scan requiring 90 sec for acquisition. **Figure 25–1A** is a 5-mm slice acquired at 1.5 T. **Figures 25–1B**, **25–1C**, and **25–1D** are from the 3 T MR unit with 5-mm, 2.5-mm, and 1-mm slice thickness, respectively.

Slice thickness in MR has decreased steadily since its clinical introduction. In the early 1980s, 10 mm was the standard slice thickness for brain imaging. With time, as magnets were introduced with higher field strengths, slice thickness decreased to 7 mm and then eventually to 5 mm. The latter represents the current standard for brain imaging at 1.5 T. With the improved SNR at 3 T, it is possible to further reduce slice thickness with preservation of image quality.

The SNR for the four scans in **Fig. 25–1**, from region-of-interest measurements in white matter, was (1.5 T) 21 and (3 T) 63, 29, and 15. As expected, there is a substantial improvement in SNR at 3 T, when slice thickness is held constant—with the 5-mm section at 1.5 T having an SNR of 21 and that at 3 T an SNR of 63. Theoretically, if all factors were held exactly constant, there should not be more than a twofold improvement in SNR at 3 T. In the images shown, the SNR at 3 T is similar to that at 1.5 T when using half the slice thickness [(**A**) versus (**C**)]. However, as one can see in this case, the SNR of the 1.5 T image actually falls between that of the 2.5-mm and 1-mm images at 3 T. Looking at this from a strict visual perspective, the "graininess" of the 5-mm 1.5 T image (**A**) is between that of the 2.5-mm (**C**) and 1-mm (**D**) sections at 3 T. The improvement beyond what is expected (a factor of two in SNR at 3 T) likely represents further hardware/software optimization on the 3 T system.

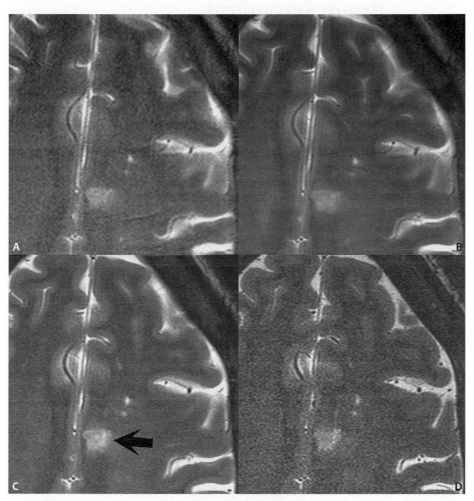

Figure 25–1

Imaging with thinner slices would not have been feasible without the advent of PACS and the filmless radiology department. As more institutions acquire 3 T systems, it seems clear that the slice thickness for routine brain imaging will continue to decrease from the current 5-mm standard to a lower number, likely 3 to 4 mm. This will give the reader a combination of improved image quality (less partial volume imaging), increased structural detail, and improved lesion detectability (for very small lesions). The current standard at our institution for a screening brain exam at 3 T, as previously noted, is 3 mm.

26 Brain: Screening

Val M. Runge and Robert S. Case

Three-tesla MR imaging offers unparalleled image quality for routine clinical brain MR, and specifically as illustrated in **Fig. 26–1** for imaging of brain infarction. We have currently adopted an approach, due to our large number of in-patients, that keeps scan times below 2 min for each scan sequence using 2D imaging with an in-plane resolution similar to that used at 1. 5 T—but with a 3-mm slice thickness as opposed to 5 mm.

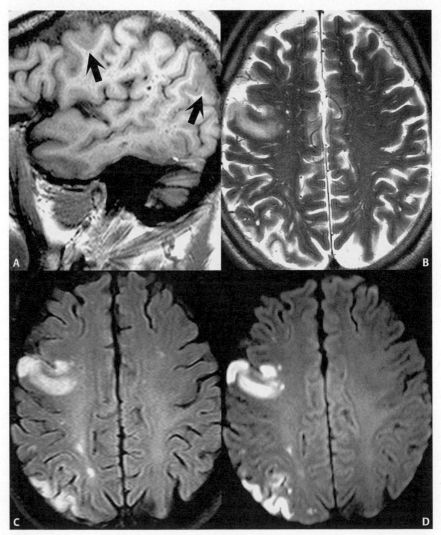

Figure 26–1

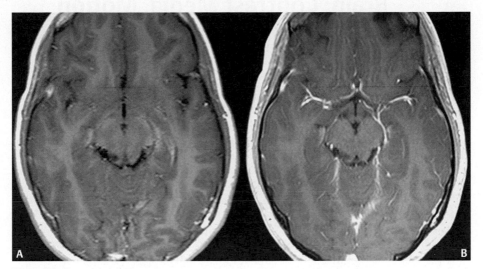

Figure 26–2

The images in **Fig. 26–1** are from a patient with an early subacute cortical infarct (middle cerebral artery and watershed distribution) and illustrate the four scans that we now acquire as our routine screening exam. A 3-mm 2D short TE spoiled GRE sagittal T1-weighted scan **(A)** is first acquired, with an acquisition time of 1:16 min:sec. Note the excellent gray-white matter differentiation on this scan, together with good visualization of cortical edema (black arrows) due to the infarct. Axial scans are subsequently acquired, all also with a 3-mm slice thickness, employing **(B)** FSE T2-weighted, **(C)** FLAIR, and **(D)** diffusion-weighted scans, with acquisition times of 1:32, 2:08, and 1:23, respectively. Including the localizer, the entire acquisition time for this screening exam is 6:42 min:sec. This represents a reduction in scan time of 40% as compared with our routine exam at 1.5 T, despite the reduction in slice thickness from 5 mm to 3 mm. 3 T MR imaging also makes possible for the first time acquisition of high-resolution diffusion-weighted scans, to be discussed in depth subsequently. This scan is acquired with a true 256^2 matrix, requiring an acquisition time of 2:23, and is illustrated in **Fig. 26–1D**, as opposed to the standard lower-resolution scan.

With regard to T1-weighted imaging of the brain, we advocate use of a short in-phase TE (2.4 msec) 2D spoiled GRE sequence, discussed in further depth in the brain neoplasia cases. The short TE (2.4 msec) limits flow-related and susceptibility artifacts. In **Fig. 26–2**, a T1-FLAIR is compared with the short TE scan in a patient with a small nonenhancing tectal lesion. Both scans are postcontrast. The T1-FLAIR required 3:09 min:sec for acquisition, using a 5-mm section, compared with 1:05 min:sec for the short TE scan, using a 3-mm section. The short TE sequence is robust and does not experience significant SAR limitations, poor tissue contrast, or accentuated motion artifacts as can be encountered with SE or FLAIR T1-weighted imaging at 3 T. Comparing directly T1-weighted SE imaging at 1.5 T and the short TE scan at 3 T, the latter offers superior SNR and CNR with reduced motion artifacts and scan time.

27 Brain: Contrast Media, Motion
Val M. Runge and Jonmenjoy Biswas

Contrast enhancement of brain lesions using the gadolinium chelates at 3 T is substantially improved when compared with 1. 5 T. In **Fig. 27–1**, coronal images (in a ratglioma model) acquired 1 min after MultiHance (Bracco Research SA, Plan-les-Ouates, Geneva, Switzerland) administration (standard dose) are compared at (A) 1.5 and (B) 3 T. Visually, there is nearly a doubling of lesion enhancement at 3 T. In **Fig. 27–2**, lesion CNR, a quantitative measure of lesion enhancement, is depicted for different time points postcontrast using an extracellular gadolinium chelate (ProHance) at both 3 T and 1.5 T, again with identical scan techniques. CNR at 3 T is consistently greater than that at 1.5 T for each time point, with the percent increase varying from 101 to 137%. Clinical results at 3 T will show somewhat less than this degree of increase. In the results cited, bandwidth was not adjusted for field strength, and SE as opposed to the short TE GRE technique was employed. Each factor by itself has a negative effect in the range of 20%.

Motion, regardless of origin, does in general cause greater artifacts at 3 T as opposed to 1.5 T. A large middle cranial fossa arachnoid cyst is illustrated in **Fig. 27–3** at (A) 1.5 and (B) 3 T, using similar scan techniques. Note the greater nonuniformity of signal intensity within the cyst at 3 T due to subtle motion therein. Likewise, arterial and venous pulsation artifacts, and ghosts due to patient movement, are typically greater at 3 T.

Attention to details of scan technique can markedly reduce motion-related artifacts at 3 T. Advances in sequence design are also affecting this area. Alternatives are available as well, in particular for gross patient motion, including fast scan techniques (discussed later) and BLADE. In **Fig. 27–4 (A, D, G)**, conventional FSE images are compared with images acquired using a propeller (BLADE) type acquisition scheme (B, E, H) without and (C, F, I) with motion correction. The techniques illustrated include (A to C) T1-weighted FLAIR, (D to F) FLAIR, and (G to I) T2-weighted FSE. The conventional images (A, D, G) are markedly degraded by

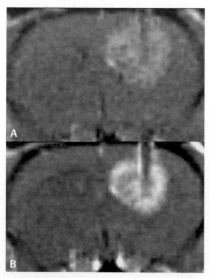

Figure 27–1

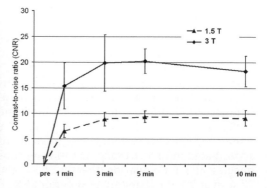

Figure 27–2

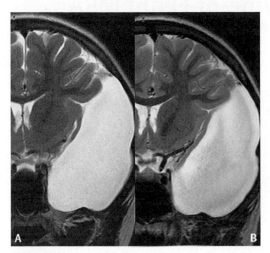

motion, with the volunteer instructed to move continuously during the scan (in-plane). Due to the radial nature of the propeller type acquisition scheme, pulsation and motion artifacts are expressed in a more benign way; thus, even without motion correction, the scans (**B, E, H**) are markedly improved. Application of motion correction results in a further improvement in image quality (**C, F, I**). Scan times were held constant for the FSE versus BLADE comparisons.

Figure 27–3

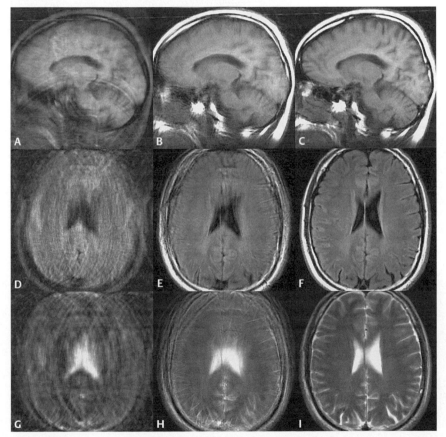

Figure 27–4

28 Brain: 3D Time-of-Flight MRA

Val M. Runge and Harold L. Sonnier

Figure 28–1 presents a maximum intensity projection (MIP) image from a 3D time-of-flight (TOF) MR angiogram obtained at 3 T in a patient with a small (<3 mm) left ophthalmic artery aneurysm. Not well seen on the MIP image, but clearly visible on source images, is the normal ophthalmic artery originating from the aneurysm. 3 T MR imaging represents a major step forward in image quality for TOF MR angiography (MRA). This is nowhere more evident than in 3D TOF MRA

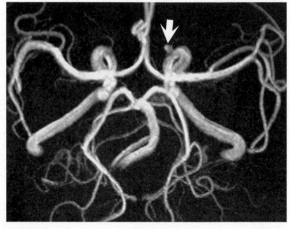

Figure 28–1

of the circle of Willis. The lengthening of T1 at 3 T is in part responsible for this marked improvement. TOF contrast is based on the visualization of fresh unsaturated blood, which has not yet reached steady state, flowing into the excitation volume. The rate at which the flow of blood approaches steady state is based on TR and flip angle, from a pulse sequence perspective, and T1 and flow characteristics from a physiological perspective. At 3 T, T1 lengthening results in the steady-state signal level for stationary tissue being reduced, providing greater vessel contrast. This lessens the need for the use of magnetization transfer, permitting the use of shorter TRs and lower flip angles to increase depth penetration.

    Figure 28–2 presents targeted MIP images of a multilobed 8-mm middle cerebral artery (MCA) aneurysm, arising from the M1 segment, acquired at **(A)** 1.5 and **(B)** 3 T. In this case, the greater signal available at 3 T has been used in part to improve spatial resolution. Two small branch vessels (arrows) originate from the aneurysm, a critical

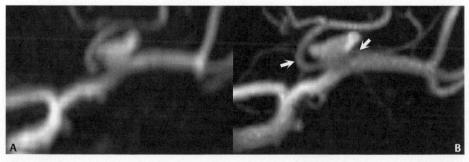

Figure 28–2

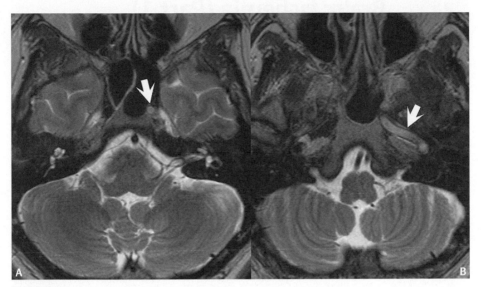

Figure 28–3

imaging finding, with the origin of the larger vessel not depicted and the smaller vessel itself not even evident on the 1.5 T scan. Voxel dimensions were $0.8 \times 0.8 \times 1$ mm^3 at 1.5 T and $0.4 \times 0.4 \times 0.4$ mm^3 at 3 T, with scan times of 6:08 and 8:28 min:sec, respectively.

T2-weighted axial images presented in **Fig. 28–3** reveal abnormal high signal intensity within the left petrous portion of the internal carotid artery (arrows). This is consistent with either very slow flow or occlusion. An MIP projection of the 3D TOF MRA of the circle of Willis **(Fig. 28–4)** demonstrates occlusion of the petrous and cavernous portions of the left internal carotid artery, with only the carotid terminus (arrow) visualized. The left MCA is supplied via collateral flow from the anterior and left posterior communicating arteries. Duplex ultrasound confirmed the absence of flow in the left internal carotid artery. Note the reduced signal intensity of the left middle cerebral artery and its branches, relative to the normal right side, due to slow flow. The excellent visualization of both small arteries and distal branching vessels, illustrated in both this and previous figures, is a consistent result with 3D TOF MRA at 3 T.

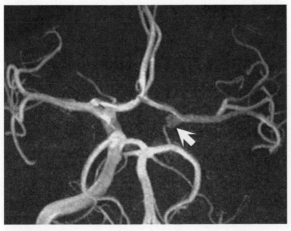

Figure 28–4

29 Brain: Ischemia (Part 1)

Val M. Runge and Robert S. Case

3 T MR imaging offers for the first time the ability to do high in-plane resolution, as well as thin section, diffusion-weighted imaging (DWI), as illustrated in **Figs. 29–1**, **29–2**, and **29–3**. The images in **Figs. 29–1** and **29–2** are from a 57-year-old man with a history of hypertension who presented with right-sided facial droop together with right-sided upper and lower extremity weakness. An early subacute infarct is noted involving the left posterior periventricular white matter extending to involve the adjacent lentiform nucleus. The images in **Fig. 29–3** are from a 73-year-old man who presented to the emergency department with left arm weakness and unsteadiness. Multiple early subacute infarcts are noted in the right MCA as well as right MCA/PCA (posterior cerebral artery) watershed distributions. **Figures 29–1A** and **29–3A** were obtained at 1.5 T

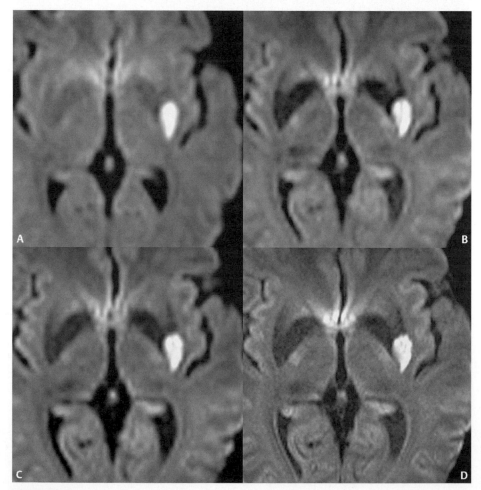

Figure 29–1

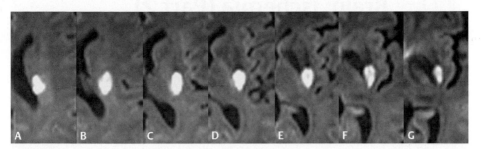

Figure 29–2

(using a 5-mm slice thickness) with the remainder of the images acquired at 3 T. **Figures 29–1B** and **29–1C** illustrate 5-mm- and 2.5-mm-thick sections at 3 T. **Figures 29–1D** and **29–3B** are high-resolution diffusion-weighted images acquired at 3 T using a 256 × 256 matrix (with an in-plane resolution of 0.9 × 0.9 mm^2 as compared with 1.9 × 1.9 mm^2 for the other scans). **Figure 29–2** illustrates multislice 2.5-mm DWI covering the craniocaudal extent of the infarct.

These figures show applications of DWI that have not been possible at 1.5 T. Thin-section DWI has the same benefits as those of thin-section T1- and T2-weighted imaging, described elsewhere in the "Brain: Ischemia" cases, including improved anatomic detail and lesion detectability. High in-plane resolution DWI also have not been clinically feasible at 1.5 T due to SNR limitations. These can be easily performed at 3 T. The scan time is longer for high-resolution DWI at 3 T, 2:23 min:sec in this instance. This compares with a scan time of 1:23 min:sec for the 3-mm 128 × 128 matrix images that we currently employ on every patient. The high-resolution DWI scan has substantially improved image detail compared with the standard exam. The margins of the abnormalities are more distinct and the smaller punctate areas of diffusion abnormality better seen (**Fig. 29–3B**). Using thinner section and high in-plane resolution DWI, both of which can be performed at 3 T, improves overall image quality and offers the possibility of improved detection of smaller infarcts (as illustrated in subsequent cases).

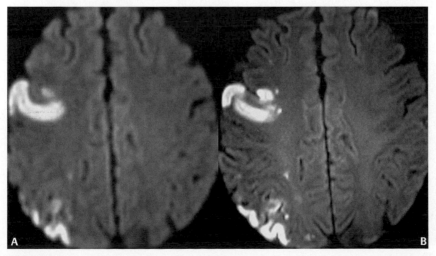

Figure 29–3

30 Brain: Ischemia (Part 2)
Val M. Runge and Harold L. Sonnier

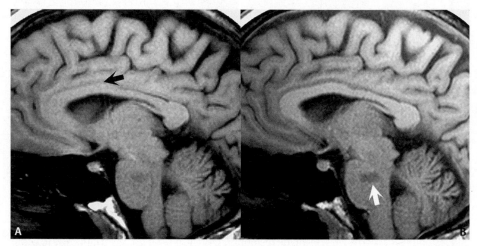

Figure 30–1

The images in **Figs. 30–1** and **30–2** are from a 57-year-old diabetic with a 1-day history of unsteadiness. Midline sagittal T1-weighted images (**Fig. 30–1**) depict an early subacute pontine infarct (white arrow) at (**A**) 1.5 T and (**B**) 3 T. Two-dimensional SE technique was employed at 1.5 T with TR/TE = 550/12, a slice thickness of 5 mm, and

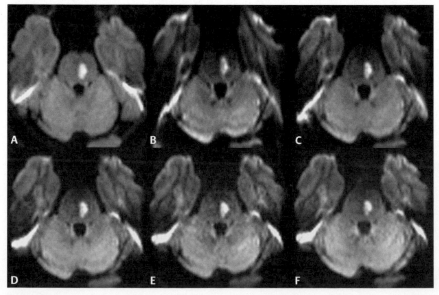

Figure 30–2

a scan time of 2:55 min:sec. Two-dimensional GRE technique was employed at 3 T with TR/TE/tip angle = 440/2.4/90 degrees, a parallel-imaging factor of two, a slice thickness of 3 mm, and a scan time of 1 min 15 sec. Gray-white matter contrast is similar between the two scans. The 1.5 T scan demonstrates a prominent ghost (black arrow), with the 3 T scan artifact-free. The improved depiction of the pontine infarct at 3 T is largely due to less partial volume imaging (3- versus 5-mm slice thickness).

One current negative factor for 3 T is the increase in bulk susceptibility artifact (versus 1.5 T), because the influence of magnetic susceptibility scales linearly with field strength. This is particularly evident in DWI. Parallel imaging currently plays an important role in decreasing the degree of artifact, with other possible solutions including multishot echo planar imaging (EPI) currently in development. **Figure 30–2A** is a diffusion-weighted image at 1.5 T (with a parallel-imaging factor of 2, and 3 averages), whereas the remaining images are from 3 T. **Figure 30–2B** is without parallel imaging, and **Figs. 30–2C** to **30–2F** are with parallel-imaging factors and averages of **(C)** 2, 2, **(D)** 3, 3, **(E)** 4, 4, and **(F)** 4, 8. With each increment in parallel-imaging factor, the depiction of the pons—and specifically the left pontine infarct—is improved. The degree of bulk susceptibility artifact in this region is variable from patient to patient at 3 T, with the example presented being the extreme in degree of distortion that can be seen.

The images in **Fig. 30–3** are from a 54-year-old diabetic with a 1-day history of ataxia. A small, early subacute right lateral medullary infarct is noted (arrows). In **Fig. 30–3, (A)** 5-mm 1.5 T and **(B)** 3-mm 3 T T2-weighted images are presented together with **(C)** 1.5 T and **(D)** high-resolution (256 × 256) 3 T DWI. This small medullary infarct is much better seen on the thin-section T2-weighted image at 3 T and is also more clearly visualized on the high-resolution DWI at 3 T. Clearly illustrated is the improved lesion detectability at 3 T secondary to improved SNR, permitting thinner section imaging with less volume averaging and higher in-plane resolution (on DWI).

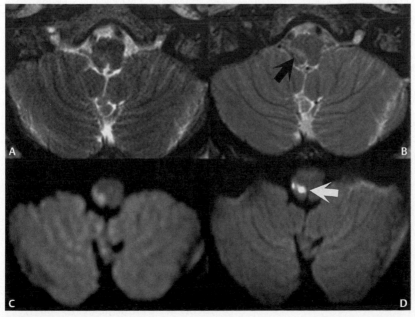

Figure 30–3

31 Brain: Ischemia (Part 3)

Val M. Runge

Presented in **Fig. 31–1** are 3-mm axial **(A)** FLAIR, **(B)** FSE T2-weighted, and **(C)** DWI images (with scan times of 1:30, 1:56, and 1:23 min:sec) from the 3 T scan of a 50-year-old male who presented to the emergency room with weakness involving the right half of the body, clumsiness, and slurred speech 12 hours prior to the MR exam. Abnormal high signal intensity is seen on DWI near the interface between the lateral thalamus and posterior limb of the internal capsule on the left. The lesion was seen on three adjacent slices, an advantage of thin-section imaging, easing lesion recognition and diagnosis. On FLAIR and T2-weighted images, only a very subtle abnormal increase in signal intensity is visualized. Cytotoxic edema occurs within minutes of an ischemic event and

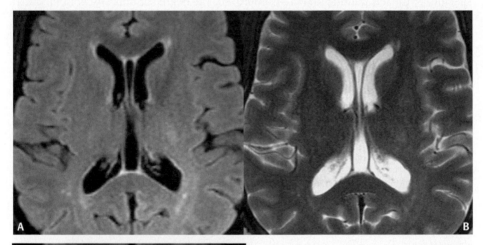

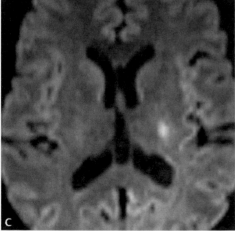

is visualized on MR as restricted diffusion (high signal intensity on DWI). Vasogenic edema develops subsequently and is depicted on T2-weighted scans as abnormal high signal intensity. T2-weighted images are often normal within the first 8 hours after infarction, with the lesion becoming progressively hyperintense from 8 to 24 hours. Ninety percent of lesions will have abnormal high signal intensity on T2-weighted scans by 24 hours. The acute (<24 hours) lacunar infarct in this patient thus demonstrates by MR a classic appearance, with predominantly cytoxic edema and little if any vasogenic edema at this time point (12 hours).

Figure 31–1

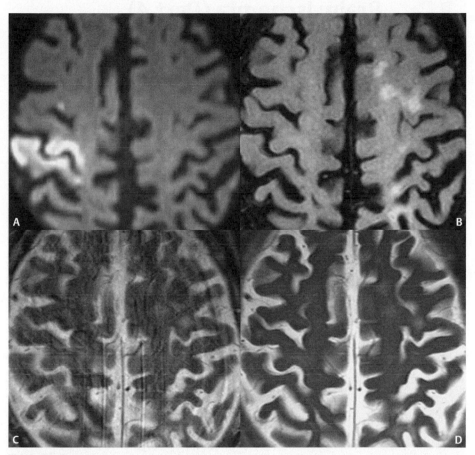

Figure 31–2

Presented in **Fig. 31–2** are 3-mm axial **(A)** DWI, **(B)** FLAIR, **(C)** FSE, and **(D)** HASTE T2-weighted images in an 80-year-old man with an acute (<24 hours) infarct. Much like imaging findings in **Fig. 31–1**, an abnormality is noted on DWI with little corresponding change on T2-weighted images. Abnormal high signal intensity is seen in the right pre- and postcentral gyrus on DWI, reflecting cytotoxic edema. Little to no abnormality is noted in the corresponding location on T2-weighted scans. This case also illustrates the use at 3 T of HASTE as an alternative to FSE T2-weighted imaging in uncooperative patients. Motion artifact in this instance substantially degrades **(C)** the FSE T2-weighted scan. The acquisition time for this scan was 1:42 min:sec, with the scan being 2D multislice in type. **(D)** The HASTE scan is acquired in single-slice mode, with a scan time of 0.6 sec per slice, markedly limiting artifacts due to patient motion. Also noted on the scans in this individual is abnormal high signal intensity within the white matter of the centrum semiovale on the left, best seen on FLAIR, the residual of a chronic left MCA distribution infarct.

32 Brain: Ischemia (Part 4)

Val M. Runge and Robert S. Case

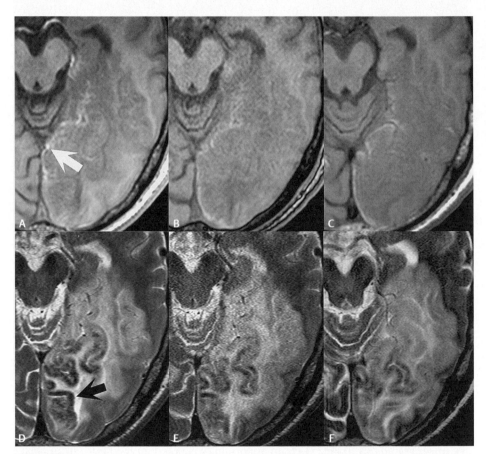

Figure 32–1

Figures **32–1** and **32–2** are from the exam of an 83-year-old hypertensive man with atrial fibrillation who presented with a 1-week history of confusion and visual disturbances. There is a large left posterior cerebral artery, early subacute infarct, which demonstrates both petechial methemoglobin (white arrow) and deoxyhemoglobin (black arrow). **Figures 32–1A** and **32–1B** were acquired using the identical short TE 2D spoiled GRE sequence (with a slice thickness of

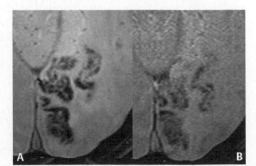

Figure 32–2

3 mm) but at **(A)** 3 T as opposed to **(B)** 1.5 T. The bandwidth, together with all other sequence parameters, has been held constant. The graininess of the 1.5 T image reflects the lower SNR. **Figure 32–1C** is a routine 5-mm scan from the 1.5 T using SE technique. The scan times were 1:05, 1:05, and 4:49 min:sec, respectively. **Figures 32–1D** to **32–1F** present a similar comparison for T2-weighted FSE imaging. **Figures 32–1D** and **32–1E** were acquired using identical scan technique (with a slice thickness of 3 mm) but at **(D)** 3 T as opposed to **(E)** 1.5 T. The difference in SNR between the images again primarily reflects the difference in field strength. **Figure 32–1F** is a routine 5-mm T2-weighted scan from 1.5 T using FSE technique and with the bandwidth optimized for 1.5 T. The scan times were 1:12, 1:12, and 1:29 min:sec, respectively. Note in both instances (T1- and T2-weighted scans) that the 3-mm 3 T images have similar to slightly improved SNR compared with the standard 5-mm scans at 1.5 T. **Figure 32–2** compares GRE images at **(A)** 3 T to that at **(B)** 1.5 T in the same patient, again using identical imaging parameters. Note the markedly increased susceptibility effect at 3 T as compared with 1.5 T, and thus the improved visualization of deoxyhemoglobin in this subacute infarct. This effect can also be appreciated, albeit to a lesser extent, in comparing the FSE T2-weighted images at 3 and 1.5 T.

A single small focus of gliosis is noted on a 1.5 T FLAIR exam **(Fig. 32–3A)**. The equivalent level is shown at 3 T **(C)**, but using a 3-mm as opposed to 5-mm slice thickness, with the same small gliotic lesion noted (white arrow). Inspection of the slices above and below this level on the 3 T exam **(B, D)** reveal additional foci of gliosis (black arrows) not seen on adjacent slices at 1.5 T. It should be kept in mind that when moving to thinner sections at 3 T, visualization of small punctate lesions will typically be improved, due to less partial volume imaging, leading to chronic small vessel white ischemic disease often appearing more prominent, as in this example.

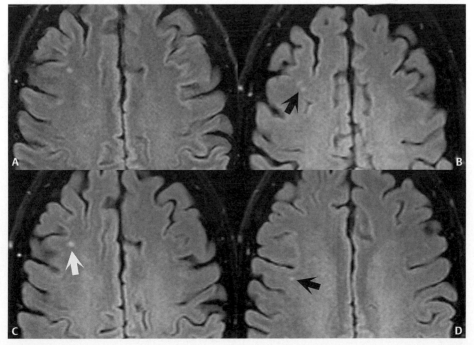

Figure 32–3

33 Brain: Infection/Inflammation
Val M. Runge

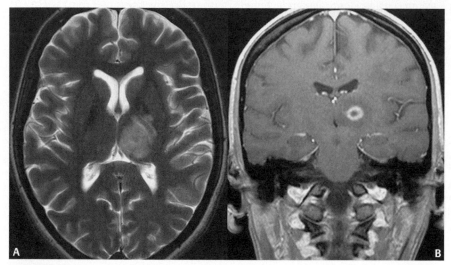

Figure 33–1

Figure 33–1 presents axial T2- and coronal postcontrast T1-weighted images from a 27-year-old patient with AIDS and a ring-enhancing toxoplasmosis lesion, with accompanying edema, in the left thalamus. **Figure 33–2** presents axial postcontrast T1-weighted images in a patient with cryptococcal meningitis. Multiple areas of focal leptomeningeal enhancement are noted (arrows), including the 7th and 8th cranial nerve complex within the internal auditory canals bilaterally. Compared with 1.5 T, 3 T

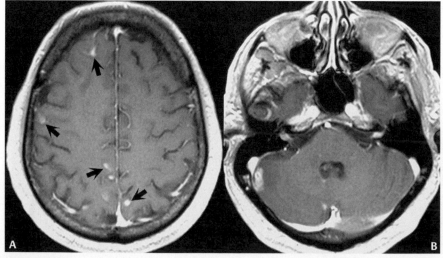

Figure 33–2

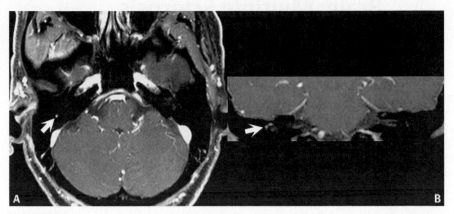

Figure 33–3

MR imaging holds definite advantages in the evaluation of brain infection. Short scan times and high sensitivity to contrast enhancement are important in a patient population prone to motion and with lesions often poorly enhancing, due to immunosuppression (or intrinsically, as with leptomeningeal disease).

Figure 33–3 presents axial and coronal 2-mm postcontrast T1-weighted images with fat saturation (3:42 scan time, short TE 2D GRE technique) in a 51-year-old patient with Bell's palsy on the right. The scan was performed to exclude other underlying disease. Demonstration of enhancement of the 7th cranial nerve (arrows), due to inflammation with Bell's palsy, in our experience is markedly improved at 3 T. This is not surprising given the access to high SNR thin-section imaging and improved contrast sensitivity.

Figure 33–4 presents axial 3-mm T2- and postcontrast T1-weighted images demonstrating edema and enhancement of the left optic nerve in a 41-year-old female with optic neuritis. Vision improved dramatically after empirical therapy with steroids. Thin-section imaging (3 mm) and short scan times (1:12 and 0:51 min:sec, respectively, in this instance) in routine screening exams at 3 T have dramatically improved depiction of the globe and intraorbital optic nerve, due to decreased partial volume imaging and less time for inadvertent ocular motion. The impact has been greatest for demonstration of optic nerve lesions and ocular pathology, the latter including principally primary and secondary neoplastic lesions.

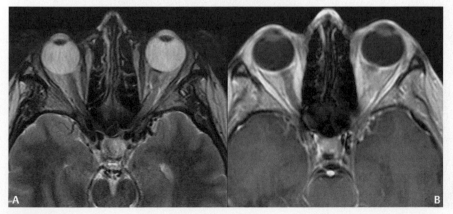

Figure 33–4

34 Brain: Multiple Sclerosis
Val M. Runge

Figure 34–1 presents **(A, B)** axial T2- and **(C, D)** axial and sagittal T1-weighted images in a 39-year-old woman with a 5-year history of relapsing-remitting multiple sclerosis (MS). **(A, C, D)** Multiple punctate periventricular lesions are noted, together with **(B)** a lesion (arrow) within the left inferior cerebellar peduncle. Thin-section imaging improves depiction of both chronic (as in this case) and active lesions. **Figure 34–2** presents 3-mm diffusion (DWI) and T2-weighted axial images in a 29-year-old woman with relapsing-remitting MS and a 5-day history of diplopia, vertigo, and unsteady gait. Multiple punctate, both large and small, white matter lesions are noted. On DWI, many of the lesions are high signal intensity, consistent with their acute nature (as also demonstrated on postcontrast scans, not shown). As illustrated, 3 mm imaging has markedly improved depiction of small lesions on DWI. **Fig. 34–3** presents axial FLAIR and postcontrast T1-weighted images from the same patient, at a higher level. A large enhancing supraventricular lesion is noted on both scans. Identified only on the postcontrast scan (arrow, **B**) is a small punctate enhancing MS plaque. New lesions may be seen first only due to contrast enhancement,

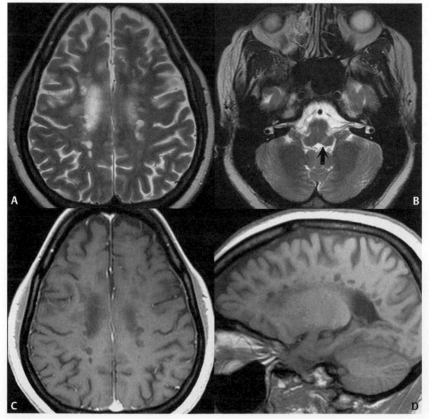

Figure 34–1

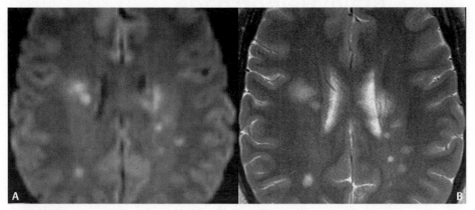

Figure 34–2

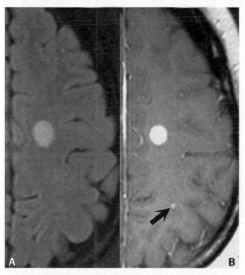

Figure 34–3

with detection of small such lesions, as with metastatic disease (discussed in later cases), markedly improved at 3 T due to higher SNR (leading to higher CNR) and the use of thin sections.

Figure 34–4 presents axial FLAIR images obtained at **(A)** 1.5 and **(B)** 3 T in a 46-year-old woman with a 16-year history of relapsing remitting MS. Slice thickness and scan time were respectively **(A)** 5 mm, 3:09 and **(B)** 2.5 mm, 1:57. The lesions are better delineated at 3 T, with several small lesions only noted on the 3 T exam. Published studies comparing 1.5 and 3 T in the evaluation of MS have demonstrated that scans at 3 T show a substantial increase in number of enhancing lesions, enhancing lesion volume, and plaque burden (total lesion volume).

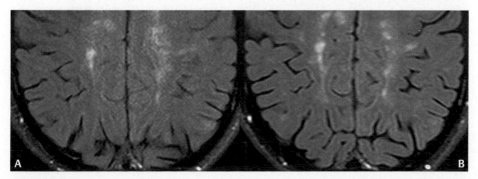

Figure 34–4

35 Brain: Hemorrhage

Val M. Runge

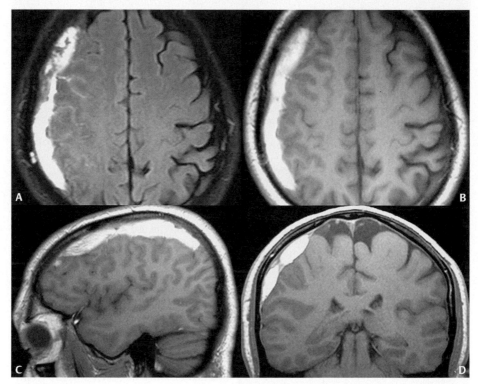

Figure 35–1

The imaging characteristics of hemorrhage differ little at 3 T from those at 1.5 T, other than the improved sensitivity to blood products that exhibit T2* effects (deoxyhemoglobin,

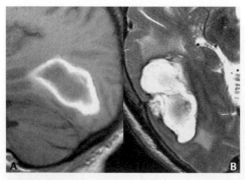

Figure 35–2

intracellular methemoglobin, and hemosiderin). **Figure 35–1** presents **(A)** axial FLAIR and **(B)** axial, **(C)** sagittal, and **(D)** coronal T1-weighted scans in a young man with a subacute, extracellular methemoglobin subdural hematoma (high signal intensity on both T1- and T2-weighted scans). Note the exquisite depiction of the adjacent sulcal effacement. **Figure 35–2** presents **(A)** sagittal T1- and **(B)** axial T2-weighted images from the exam of an 88-year-old woman with a right parietal hematoma, 2 weeks in age. The images in **Fig. 35–2** are 3 mm

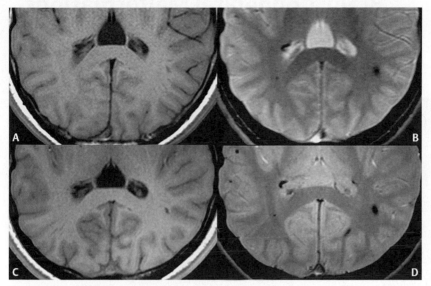

Figure 35–3

in slice thickness, with scan times of 1:15 and 1:30. The periphery of the hematoma is composed of extracellular methemoglobin. Hemosiderin is likely already present at the interface between the hematoma and surrounding brain, leading to the thin rim of low signal intensity on the T2-weighted scan.

Figures 35–3 and **Fig. 35–4** present scans from a patient with multiple cavernous malformations, imaged at both 1.5 T (**Figs. 35–3A, 35–3B,** and **Fig. 35–4A**) and 3 T (**Fig. 35–3C, 35–3D,** and **Fig. 35–4B**). In **Fig. 35–3, (A, C)** T1-weighted and **(B, D)** GRE T2-weighted scans are compared. In **Fig. 35–4,** T2-weighted FSE scans are compared. The images at 1.5 T were 5 mm in slice thickness, as compared with 3 mm at 3 T. Scan times were comparable at 1.5 versus 3 T, with the exception that the T1-weighted scan required 3:09 (min:sec) at 1.5 T versus 1:05 at 3 T. Note the improved depiction of the many lesions in this patient at 3 T, due to a combination of the decreased slice thickness (reduced partial volume effect) together with the increased sensitivity to susceptibility effects. Examining each sequence pair (specifically the respective scans at 1.5 and 3 T), the lesions are best visualized at 3 T, with low signal intensity due to their hemosiderin content. The images at 1.5 T also appear slightly "grainy," due to lower SNR.

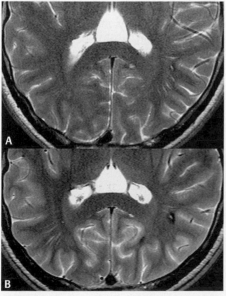

Figure 35–4

36 Brain: Congenital Malformations
Val M. Runge

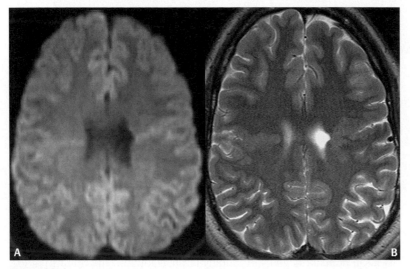

Figure 36–1

3 T should emerge long-term as the field strength of choice for MR imaging of congenital malformations, due to improved high-resolution, thin-section imaging capabilities. The latter can lead to a marked improvement in depiction of many of these entities. Schizencephaly is characterized by clefts extending from the cortical pial surface to the ventricle, lined by nodular (polymicrogyric) gray matter. Thin-section (3 mm) imaging improves recognition of the bilateral "closed-lip" defects noted in **Fig. 36–1** on both **(A)** DWI and **(B)** T2-weighted scans. The mild deformity of the left lateral ventricle "points" to the cleft in this 18-year-old presenting with seizures.

Figure 36–2 illustrates small bilateral frontal cortical/subcortical tubers in a patient with seizures and tuberous sclerosis. Thin-section (3 mm) imaging makes possible recognition of rather small lesions (arrows) in this instance, depicted with hyperintensity on **(A)** FLAIR and hypointensity on **(B)** T1-weighted imaging (2D short TE GRE).

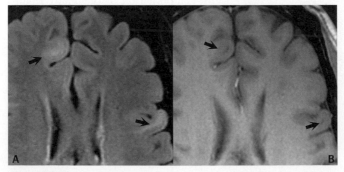

Figure 36–2

37 Brain: Toxic/Degenerative Disorders

Val M. Runge

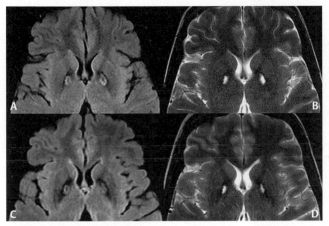

Figure 37–1

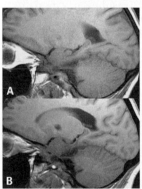

Figure 37–2

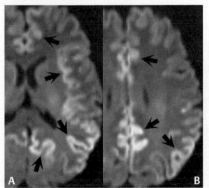

Figure 37–3

Illustrated in **Fig. 37–1** and **Fig. 37–2** is a case of carbon monoxide poisoning, from a failed suicide attempt, with bilateral chronic necrotic lesions in the globus pallidus. **Figures 37–1A, 37–1B**, and **37–2A** are at 1.5 T, and **Figs. 37–1C, 37–1D,** and **37–2B** at 3 T. FLAIR, T2-, and T1-weighed images are shown. On axial imaging at 3 T, the lesions were noted on two adjacent slices, whereas these were seen on only one axial section at 1.5 T, due to the thicker slice (5 versus 3 mm). On sagittal imaging, the lesions were well visualized only at 3 T (due to use of a 3-mm slice thickness).

Illustrated in **Fig. 37–3** on DWI at 3 T is Creutzfeldt-Jakob disease (CJD). Thin-section imaging (3 mm) with DWI at 3 T has led to markedly improved utility of this scan, in both infarction and secondary applications. In CJD, DWI has the highest sensitivity for detection of signal intensity abnormalities. Cortical (gyriform) hyperintense areas in the cerebral hemispheres are characteristic, as seen in this case (arrows). The cortical nature of disease involvement is readily evident, due largely to the reduced partial volume effects and high SNR in these scans.

38 Brain: Neoplasia—Introduction

Val M. Runge and Harold L. Sonnier

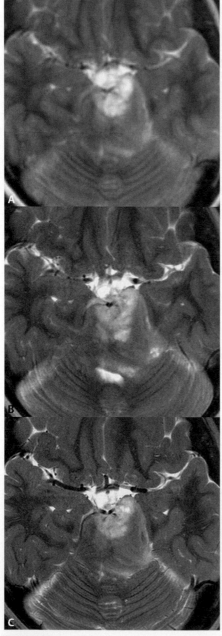

Figure 38–1

For the evaluation of brain neoplasia, in common with many other anatomic/pathologic areas, one is confronted at 3 T with the dilemma of whether to use the additional available SNR for improved spatial resolution or to decrease scan time. Often, the scan that is adopted clinically represents a compromise between the two extremes. **Figure 38–1** illustrates images from a patient with a brainstem (pontine) astrocytoma using T2-weighted FSE technique. The spectrum of scan time and resultant image quality is illustrated, with the acquisition time varying from 24 seconds to 59 seconds to 2:39 min:sec **(A to C)**. Spatial (voxel) resolution varied from $0.7 \times 0.7 \times 5$ to $0.5 \times 0.4 \times 5$ to $0.4 \times 0.4 \times 2.5$ mm³ **(A to C)**. Patients with or suspected of neoplastic disease in the brain represent a subpopulation in which inadvertent motion is often a problem in regard to scan quality. To ask such a patient to hold still—meaning moving well less than one half of a mm—for a 5-min scan with an in-plane resolution of less than 0.5×0.5 mm² and a slice thickness less than 5 mm is simply not practical. A reasonable compromise is a 3- to 5-mm slice thickness, with an in-plane resolution of greater than 0.5×0.5 mm², which due to the robust nature of FSE T2-weighted imaging at 3 T can be performed in 1 to 2 min. Except for specialty exams, such as the internal auditory canal or pituitary, the additional spatial resolution possible with a 5-min T2-weighted scan at 3 T simply does not add important clinical information, as the disease processes being examined are in themselves typically large in dimension relative to pixel resolution.

As discussed in earlier chapters, an in-phase short TE (2.4 msec) 2D GRE scan is strongly recommended for routine brain imaging at 3 T and is indeed critical for

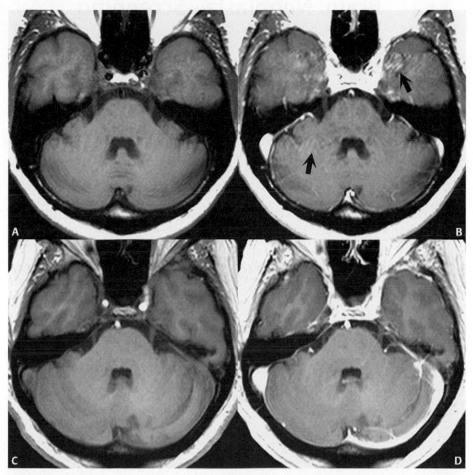

Figure 38–2

postcontrast T1-weighted imaging in brain neoplastic disease. **Figure 38–2** illustrates an age-matched comparison of **(A, C)** pre- and **(B, D)** postcontrast images acquired at 1.5 and 3 T. Scan times were 3:44 (pre) and 5:02 (post), for a 5-mm slice, at 1.5 T as compared with 1:11 (pre and post), for a 3-mm slice, at 3 T. Note the vascular pulsation artifacts on the 1.5 T study, accentuated postcontrast (arrows), despite the use of gradient moment nulling (flow compensation). No ghosting is evident on the 3 T study. Thus, despite statements in the literature to the contrary, excellent T1-weighted images of the brain can easily be acquired at 3 T by use of short TE 2D GRE technique, a critical point for tumor imaging.

39 Brain: Neoplasia—Screening

Val M. Runge and Harold L. Sonnier

Illustrated in **Fig. 39–1** are the routine T2-weighted and postcontrast T1-weighted scans acquired for screening in neoplastic disease of the brain. The images are from a 58-year-old man who presented with a 6-week history of memory and cognitive difficulties, with biopsy confirming a glioblastoma multiforme. Scan times were **(A)** 0:59, **(B)** 1:05, and **(D)** 0:51 min:sec, with the slice thickness being 3 mm for all three scans. **(B)** and **(D)** were acquired using the short TE 2D GRE approach. SE T1-weighted imaging is not recommended **(C)** for routine screening of the brain at 3 T, due to long scan times (2:20 in this instance for 5-mm sections), accentuated motion artifacts, SAR limitations, and inhomogeneity over the field of view. The latter, likely due to dielectric effects, is well illustrated in **(C)**. Note the artificial increase in brain signal intensity from

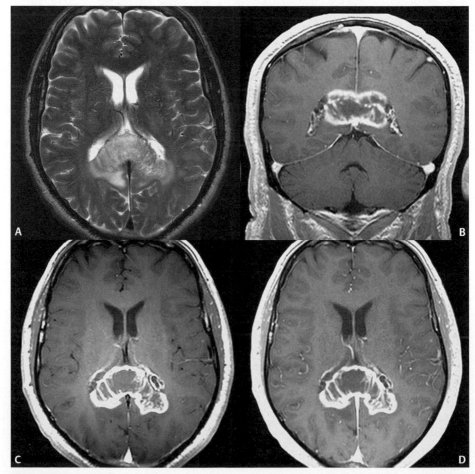

Figure 39–1

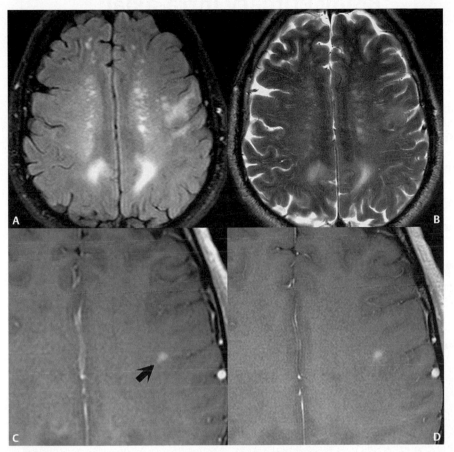

Figure 39–2

the periphery to the center of the image. With SE imaging, the cerebrospinal fluid signal intensity may also be variable from patient to patient (often slightly elevated). Care should also be exercised due to the possible short acquisition time of the postcontrast scan, as enhancement for most intra-axial lesions is maximal 5 to 10 minutes after IV gadolinium chelate injection. It is quite possible to scan too rapidly postcontrast. This can be avoided by incorporating a delay between contrast injection and initiation of the postcontrast scans. One more time-efficient alternative is to acquire the T2-weighted FSE sequence as the first scan postcontrast, as this sequence is essentially unaffected by the contrast agent, using what might otherwise be time wasted while the patient is in the scanner.

Figure 39–2 is from the same patient, but at a higher level illustrating the multifocal nature of the lesion. A second small enhancing focus (arrow), distant from the bulk of the mass in the splenium of the corpus callosum, is identified. The standard FLAIR (**A**), T2- (**B**), and T1- (**C**) weighted images acquired in routine screening are illustrated, the latter postcontrast, with scan times of 2:08, 1:32, and 0:51 (all 3 mm). Although not advocated for routine screening, a high-resolution 5:22 postcontrast T1-weighted GRE scan is also shown (**D**), with a pixel dimension of 0.5×0.5 mm^2 as compared with 0.9×0.9 mm^2 for (**C**), illustrating the anatomic detail possible at 3 T.

40 Brain: Primary Intra-axial Neoplasia

Val M. Runge and Jonmenjoy Biswas

For the evaluation of primary brain tumors, 3 T offers chiefly decreased scan time and thin-section routine imaging. In clinical practice, the decrease in scan time is not insignificant, with image quality improved overall. Scans are shorter with less time for patients to move and as a consequence a reduction in gross motion artifacts. In **Fig. 40–1**, the FLAIR and T1-weighted scans in the upper row **(A, B)** required 3:54 and 2:24 min:sec, respectively, for acquisition at 1.5 T, whereas the corresponding scans in the lower row at 3 T **(C, D)** required 1:30 and 1:15 min:sec. Depiction of the biopsy-proven oligodendroglioma (arrow) is remarkably similar on the 1.5 and 3 T scans, despite use of the short TE GRE technique for T-weighted imaging at 3 T as opposed to SE technique as employed at 1.5 T. The slice thickness at 1.5 T was 5 mm and that at 3 T was 3 mm.

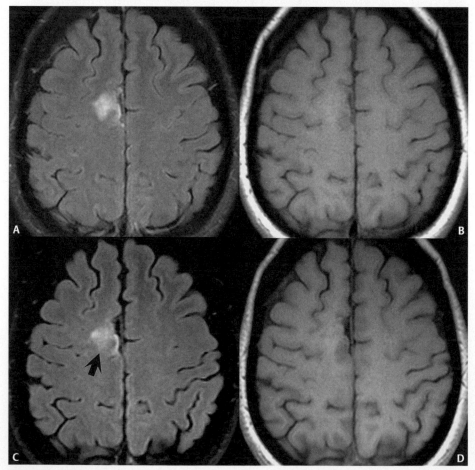

Figure 40–1

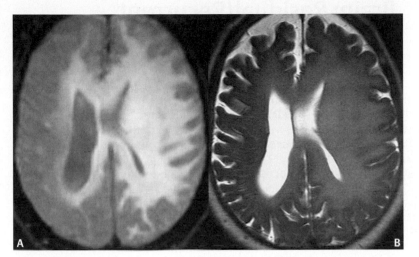

Figure 40–2

With regard to the uncooperative patient, there are multiple imaging alternatives. Two such are illustrated in **Fig. 40–2**, in a patient with gliomatosis cerebri. Echoplanar imaging **(A)** can be used to achieve FLAIR-like contrast, as illustrated, and to produce T1- or T2-weighted images. Echoplanar technique offers the advantage of a very short scan time, typically 0.06 to 0.15 sec/slice, but suffers from bulk susceptibility artifacts (increased at 3 T) and is usually acquired with a lower-resolution matrix. HASTE, illustrated in **(B),** can be used to provide T2-weighted contrast, with scan times of <1 sec/slice, but suffers from poor tissue contrast and, like echoplanar imaging, is usually acquired with reduced in-plane resolution.

A further alternative is BLADE (PROPELLER), illustrated in **Fig. 40–3** in a patient with primary lymphoma. The conventional FLAIR image is illustrated in **(A)** and the BLADE acquisition in **(B)**. BLADE combines a radial-like k-space acquisition with the potential for motion correction.

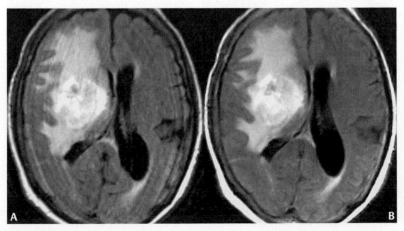

Figure 40–3

41 Brain: Residual/Recurrent Neoplasia (Part 1)

Val M. Runge

Illustrated in **Fig. 41–1** is a brainstem (pontine) glioma, in a 14-year-old, on **(A)** axial T2-weighted and postcontrast **(B to D)** axial, sagittal, and coronal T1-weighted images at 3 T. The patient has been treated with both radiation and chemotherapy. Scan times are 1:56, 1:05, 1:15, and 1:05 min:sec, with all scans 3 mm in thickness. The pixel (in plane) resolution is 0.6×0.4 mm^2 (T2) and 0.9×0.9 mm^2 (T1). The lack of pulsation artifacts postcontrast is due to use of the short TE 2D GRE technique.

There is a TE threshold for arterial and venous pulsation artifacts, with the choice of TE = 2.4 msec being in-phase at 3 T and at or just below the limit for such ghosting— thus the efficacy of the GRE scan. It has been suggested that a T1-weighted FLAIR scan is a suitable alternative to SE imaging at 3 T, with this scan implemented at some sites

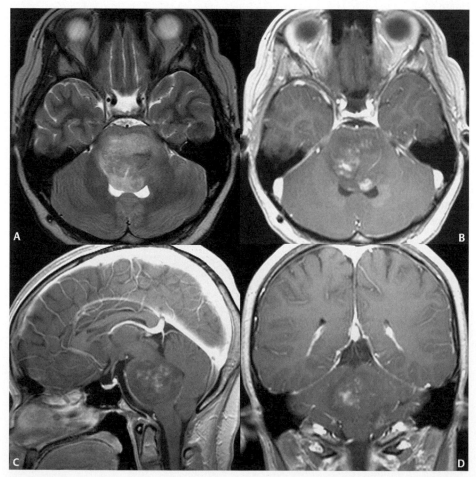

Figure 41–1

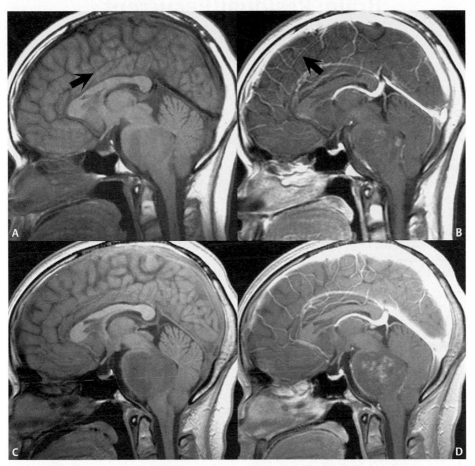

Figure 41–2

for routine clinical use. Disadvantages of the T1-weighted FLAIR scan, published in the scientific literature, include substantial arterial and venous ghosting, SAR limitations, and a long scan time. Use of this sequence is not advocated.

Sagittal T1-weighted scans **(A, C)** pre- and **(B, D)** postcontrast in the same patient are compared from **(A, B)** a 1.5 T and **(C, D)** a 3 T scanner in **Fig. 41–2**. Scan times were 1:52 and 2:32 at 1.5 T versus 1:15 and 1:15 min:sec at 3 T. A 5-mm slice thickness was used at 1.5 T compared with 3 mm at 3 T. The pixel dimensions were 1.0 to 1.1 × 0.9 mm² at 1.5 T versus 0.8 × 0.8 mm² at 3 T. Ghosting (arrows) from the superior sagittal sinus is evident on the SE images acquired at 1.5 T, both pre- and postcontrast, and absent on the short TE GRE images acquired at 3 T. Soft tissue (examine closely the cerebellum) and vascular detail is also improved on the 3 T images, likely due to the smaller voxel volume and reduced overall motion artifact.

Concern has been raised in regard to possible differences in tissue contrast on scans at 3 T as compared with 1.5 T, and the possible effect on image interpretation. Fortunately, for the brain, although pulse sequences may differ substantially, the resulting images are remarkably similar. Minor differences include greater T2* effects and on the 2D T1-weighted GRE scan the depiction of marrow (which appears with lower signal intensity).

42 Brain: Residual/Recurrent Neoplasia (Part 2)

Val M. Runge

Presented in **Fig. 42–1** are postoperative scans in a pediatric patient with a pilocytic astrocytoma (grade I). Axial T1-weighted scans **(A, C)** pre- and **(B, D)** postcontrast are compared from **(A, B)** a 1.5 T and **(C, D)** a 3 T scanner. Scan times were 3:22 (both pre- and postcontrast) at 1.5 T versus 1:05 min:sec at 3 T. The slice thickness was 5 mm at 1.5 T and 3 mm at 3 T. **(A, B)** was obtained 1 month after surgery and **(C, D)** 3 months after surgery, with no intervening therapy. The fine rim of enhancement along the right side of the cavity at 1 month corresponds with the resection margin. Three small enhancing nodular lesions (arrows), representing residual tumor, are seen on the 3 T scan, whereas only two are noted on the 1.5 T scan (with the third not seen as well on adjacent slices). At 3 T, the nodules on the left were seen on two adjacent images, with the lesion on the right on only one image. Small enhancing lesions, specifically nodular recurrence or residual (in this instance, the small nodule on the right), can be missed at 1.5 T due to the larger slice thickness and accompanying interslice gap.

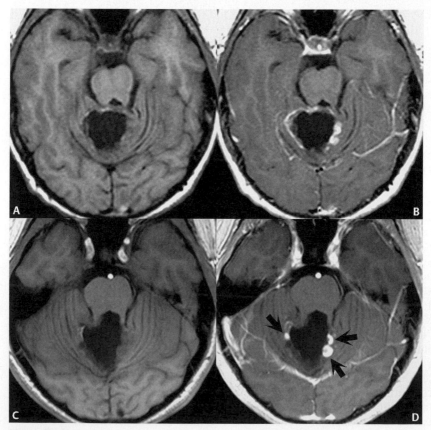

Figure 42–1

43 Brain: Metastases (Part 1)

Val M. Runge and Jonmenjoy Biswas

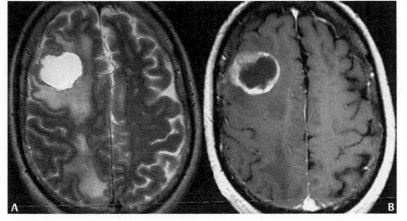

Figure 43–1

Presented in **Fig. 43–1** are **(A)** T2- and **(B)** postcontrast T1-weighted images in a patient with metastatic lung carcinoma. Scan times were 1:12 and 1:05 min:sec, respectively, with voxel dimensions of $0.6 \times 0.4 \times 3$ mm³ and $0.9 \times 0.9 \times 3$ mm³. A large centrally necrotic metastasis is visualized in the right frontal lobe, with irregular rim enhancement and substantial surrounding vasogenic edema. The appearance at 3 T is little different from that expected at 1.5 T, although the scan time is less and the slices thinner.

The potential that 3 T offers in metastatic disease of the brain is principally for improved detection of small lesions (<1 cm diameter). Note the pinpoint metastasis (arrow, **B**) visualized in **Fig. 43–2** on **(A)** pre- and **(B)** postcontrast T1-weighted GRE scans at 3 T (3-mm slice thickness), in a patient with widely metastatic transitional

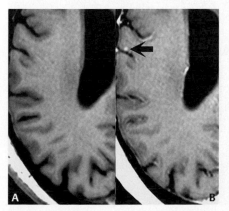

Figure 43–2

cell carcinoma. When 1.5 T and 3 T are evaluated with matched hardware and software, an improvement of ≈125% can be demonstrated with regard to detection of contrast enhancement using the gadolinium chelates at 3 T. For comparison, administering triple dose at 1.5 T leads only to ≈100% increase in lesion enhancement (and a 32% increase in number of lesions identified). The higher SNR at 3 T combined with the increased sensitivity to the gadolinium chelates should lead to improved detection of small metastases, if appropriately employed. A reduction in contrast dose, below 0.1 mmol/kg, is specifically not advised.

44 Brain: Metastases (Part 2)

Val M. Runge and Jonmenjoy Biswas

Another feature that may set 3 T apart from 1.5 T in the imaging of metastatic disease is the depiction of accompanying hemorrhage. Metastases from melanoma, small cell lung carcinoma, thyroid cancer, choriocarcinoma, and renal cell carcinoma are notable for their tendency to bleed. Given the improved visualization of T2* effects, it is possible that hemorrhage associated with a metastasis may be a more common finding at 3 T. **Fig. 44–1** illustrates a left hemispheric metastasis from non–small cell lung carcinoma with surrounding edema on **(A)** FLAIR, **(B)** T2-, **(C)** precontrast T1- and **(D)** postcontrast T1-weighted 3-mm sections at 3 T. A fine low signal intensity deoxyhemoglobin rim is best seen on the T2-weighted scan, with minimal high-signal intensity methemoglobin seen on the precontrast T1-weighted scan. The lesion demonstrates rim enhancement postcontrast.

As discussed previously, 3 T holds the potential for identification of small metastatic lesions not detected at 1.5 T, if the higher available SNR is appropriately used. **Figure 44–2** illustrates postcontrast T1-weighted images obtained at **(A)** 1.5 and **(B)** 3 T in a patient with metastatic non–small cell lung carcinoma. Two lesions (black arrows) are identified on the 3 T exam, with only one lesion seen on the 1.5 T exam. Close inspection of the images above and below that presented at 1.5 T also did not reveal the second smaller lesion. The slice thickness was 5 mm at 1.5 T and 3 mm at 3 T, with a 30% gap between slices on both exams. The smaller pinpoint metastasis

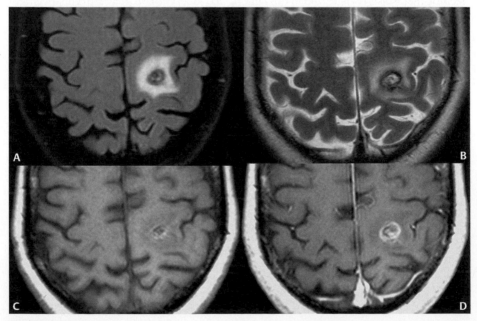

Figure 44–1

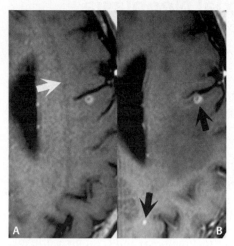

Figure 44–2

evidently lay between the thicker slices at 1.5 T and thus went undetected. A discrete ghost (white arrow) from patient motion also degrades the 1.5 T exam, with less gross motion artifact observed on average at 3 T due to the shorter scan times (in this instance, less than half that of the 1.5 T scan).

Given the improved detection of IV contrast and routine use of thin-section imaging, it is also anticipated that visualization of leptomeningeal metastatic disease will be superior at 3 T. **Figure 44–3** illustrates enhancement of the left 7th and 8th nerve complex (white arrow) within the internal auditory canal, on routine (screening) 3-mm **(A)** T2- and **(B)** postcontrast T1-weighted images, due to leptomeningeal tumor spread. Additional leptomeningeal disease involving the cerebellar folia and parenchymal metastases (not illustrated) were also noted in this patient.

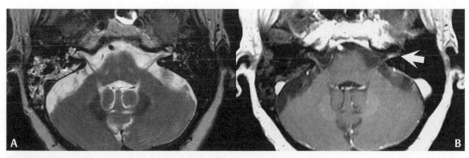

Figure 44–3

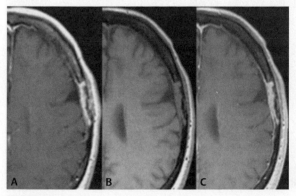

Figure 44–4

Thin-section imaging has already improved, in our experience, the detection of skull metastases, by making possible definitive visualization of smaller lesions. The short TE 2D GRE T1-weighted scan performs well in this application. A large left frontal diploic space metastasis is illustrated in **Fig. 44–4** on postcontrast 1.5 T (5 mm) and pre- and postcontrast 3 T (3 mm) T1-weighted images.

45 Brain: Extra-axial Neoplasia

Val M. Runge and Harold L. Sonnier

With regard to extra-axial neoplasia, 3 T offers, for small lesions, improved visualization, and for large lesions, improved depiction of adjacent important anatomy. Presented in **Fig. 45–1** are **(A)** pre- and **(B)** postcontrast axial 3 mm T1-weighted scans from the exam of a 45-year-old woman with a fibrous meningioma, subsequently resected. The in-plane resolution was 0.8×0.8 mm^2 and the acquisition time 1:24 min:sec for each scan. A well-defined extra-axial mass is present, smooth in contour, displacing normal brain and adjacent to the dura. There is intense homogeneous enhancement, with the exception of a central nonenhancing portion that corresponded with a large, dense calcification on CT. On the basis of the postcontrast exam, the lesion appears to invade the left transverse sinus (arrowhead). This was confirmed at surgery. Sinus invasion is not uncommon with meningiomas and is important to recognize preoperatively. Regarding surgical treatment of meningiomas, gross total resection can only be accomplished in 80% of patients, with recurrence even in this group

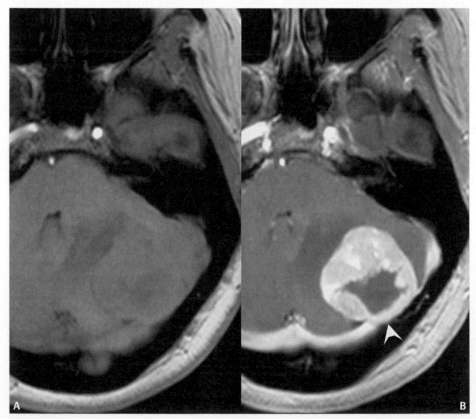

Figure 45–1

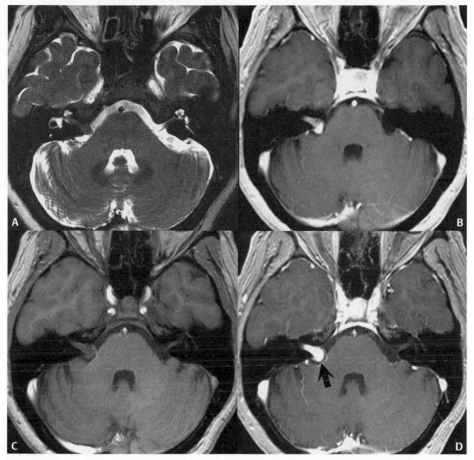

Figure 45–2

up to 30% in 10-year follow-up. This emphasizes the importance of high-quality post-operative imaging studies and thus the role of 3 T for evaluation of small residual and/or recurrent tumor—with higher routine spatial resolution than possible at 1.5 T.

Figure 45–2 illustrates a small right vestibular schwannoma with both intra- and extracanalicular components. At 3 T, 3D FSE T2-weighted imaging, illustrated in **(A)**, replaces GRE techniques such as constructive interference in a steady state (CISS) for thin-section imaging. The scan time was 5:42 min:sec in this instance, with a voxel dimension of $0.6 \times 0.6 \times 0.8$ mm^3. Although 3-mm T1-weighted imaging is fast (1:09 min:sec for acquisition of the image in **B**), thinner section, higher resolution scans—for T1-weighted imaging—are now possible on a routine basis at 3 T and pre-ferred. **(C)** Pre- and **(D)** postcontrast axial images using this approach are illustrated in **Fig. 45–2**, with voxel dimensions of $0.8 \times 0.8 \times 2$ mm^3 and a scan time of 3:15 min:sec. Note the improved depiction of this right-sided vestibular schwannoma (arrow) on post-contrast imaging with **(D)** a 2-mm slice thickness and higher in-plane resolution when compared with **(B)** 3-mm imaging. The patient was a 58-year-old woman who presented

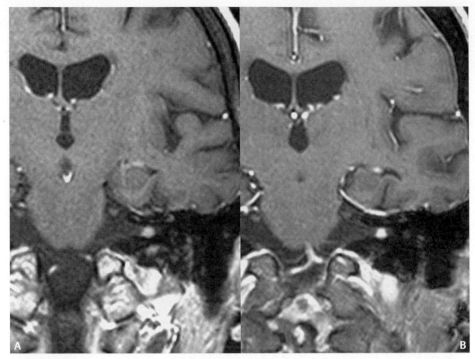

Figure 45–3

with gradual hearing loss in the right ear over the previous 6 months and increased tinnitus over the past year. Audiology demonstrated sensory neural hearing loss.

Illustrated in **Fig. 45–3**, **Fig. 45–4, and Fig. 45–5** are scans from a 76-year-old woman with sensory neural hearing loss due to a small left-sided intracanalicular vestibular

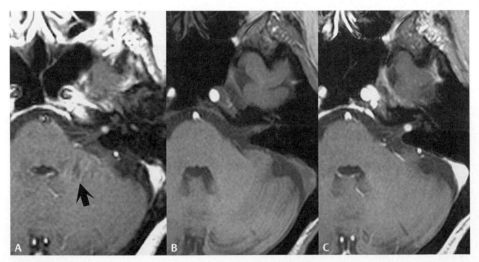

Figure 45–4

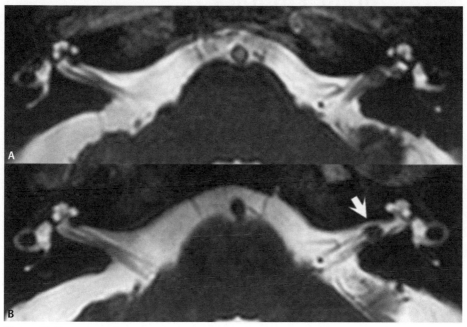

Figure 45–5

schwannoma, comparing results at 1.5 and 3 T. Postcontrast coronal T1-weighted images at **(A)** 1.5 and **(B)** 3 T are illustrated in **Fig. 45–3**: **(A)** was acquired at 1.5 T using 2D SE technique, with a scan time of 3:53 and a 3-mm slice thickness; **(B)** was acquired at 3 T using the short TE 2D spoiled GRE technique, with a scan time of 3:15 and a 2-mm slice thickness. Note the relative graininess of the 1.5 T image, reflecting the lower SNR despite the use of a thicker slice.

In **Fig. 45–4**, **(A)** an axial postcontrast T1-weighted scan at 1.5 T is compared with **(B)** pre- and **(C)** postcontrast scans at 3 T. 2D SE technique was applied at 1.5 T, with a voxel dimension of $0.9 \times 0.9 \times 3$ mm^3 and a scan time of 3:53 min:sec. 2D GRE technique was applied at 3 T, with a voxel dimension of $0.8 \times 0.8 \times 2$ mm^3 and a scan time of 3:15 min:sec. Note the prominent ghosts (arrow) on the 1.5 T image, and the absence thereof at 3 T. The images at 3 T are higher in SNR, despite the use of a smaller voxel and slightly shorter scan time, with improved depiction of this small intracanalicular lesion. A decrease in contrast dose is currently not recommended, despite the intense enhancement of vestibular schwannomas and the improved sensitivity of 3 T to the gadolinium chelates, with our experience suggesting efficacy at current dose for detection of very small lesions not previously diagnosed and more subtle nerve inflammation.

The small schwannoma present in this patient is also well demonstrated in **Fig. 45–5** on high-resolution 3 D axial T2-weighted images, albeit substantially better at 3 T: **(A)** was acquired at 1.5 T employing CISS technique with a 0.7-mm slice thickness; **(B)** was acquired at 3 T employing 3D FSE technique with an 0.8-mm slice thickness. Scan times were comparable. Depiction of the cranial nerves, together with the intracanalicular mass itself (arrow), is substantially better on the **(B)** thin-section T2-weighted scan at 3 T.

46

Brain: Pituitary

Val M. Runge

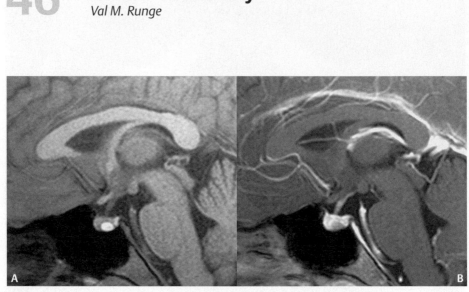

Figure 46–1

Illustrated in **Fig. 46–1** are sagittal 3-mm **(A)** pre- and **(B)** postcontrast 2D T1-weighted GRE images acquired at 3 T in a 33-year-old woman with a pituitary microadenoma (prolactinoma) previously treated with bromocriptine. The microadenoma is high-signal-intensity precontrast, due to hemorrhagic/proteinaceous content. Postcontrast, the microadenoma is slightly low signal intensity relative to the normal surrounding gland, due to the intense enhancement of the latter. Each scan required 1:23 min:sec. In-plane spatial resolution was 0.8×0.6 mm^2. No distortion of the sella floor is evident, despite the adjacent aerated sphenoid sinus and the potential for bulk susceptibility artifacts due to the use of GRE technique.

Figure 46–2 presents coronal 2-mm **(A)** pre- and **(B)** postcontrast 2D T1-weighted GRE images from a patient with a nonfunctioning pituitary macroadenoma. In-plane

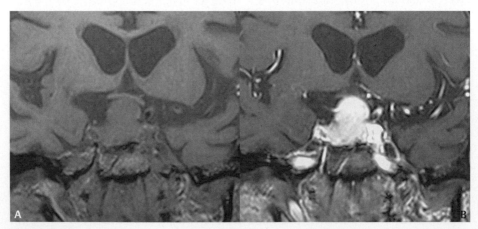

Figure 46–2

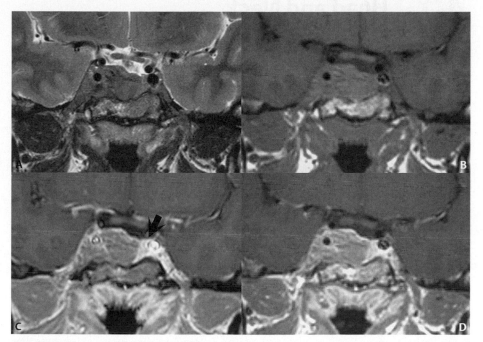

Figure 46–3

spatial resolution was 0.9×0.9 mm^2, with a scan time of 1:32 min:sec. The lesion has both intra- and suprasellar components, with some constriction at the level of the diaphragma sella. The suprasellar extent leads to compression (flattening and splaying) of the optic chiasm. There is prominent, relatively homogeneous contrast enhancement.

Despite the high quality of the images presented in the two previous figures, the short TE 2D T1-weighted GRE scan can at times be inadequate for imaging of the sella, due to bulk susceptibility artifacts. In such instances, there may be spatial distortion and/or poor visualization of soft tissue near the interface between the sella and the sphenoid sinus.

Illustrated in **Fig. 46–3** are 2D coronal 2-mm (**A**) T2-weighted FSE, (**B**) T1-weighted SE, and postcontrast T1-weighted (**C**) GRE and (**D**) SE images in a 32-year-old woman with a prolactin-secreting macroadenoma, partially treated with bromocriptine. Scan times were 5 to 6 min in each instance. Invasion of the right cavernous sinus is well depicted on all sequences, with tumor tissue circumferential to the cavernous carotid artery. The normal pituitary gland (arrow, **C**) is compressed against the left wall of the sella, adjacent to the normally enhancing cavernous sinus on that side. There is heterogeneous enhancement of tumor postcontrast, with much of the lesion demonstrating little to no enhancement (likely related to ongoing therapy). All scans demonstrate some internal morphology (structure) to the lesion. Examining closely the tumor within the right side of the sella, subtle areas of low signal intensity can be seen on T2- and T1-weighted scans precontrast, which demonstrate little enhancement. SE T1-weighted imaging is recommended at 3 T in instances where bulk susceptibility artifact markedly degrades the GRE scan (not the case in this example). Whether thin-section 3 T pituitary imaging offers a substantial advance clinically awaits further experience, although this is likely given the small structures involved.

47

Head and Neck
Val M. Runge and Jonmenjoy Biswas

Due to shorter scan times, 3 T offers improved imaging in ENT, in particular in the orbit and soft tissues of the neck. These are areas susceptible in particular to inadvertent patient motion, whether due to eye motion or swallowing. Illustrated in **Fig. 47–1**, **(A)** sagittal T1-, **(B)** axial T2-, and **(C)** pre- and **(D)** post-contrast axial T1-weighted images at 3 T reveal a left retinal detachment secondary to an ocular metastasis. The patient was a 70-year-old woman with previously resected adenocarcinoma of the gastroesophageal junction, now metastatic. The scans acquired were those used for routine brain screening [with the exception of the application of fat saturation in **(D)**], with a slice thickness of 3 mm and acquisition times of 1:15, 1:22, 2:10, and 1:45 min:sec.

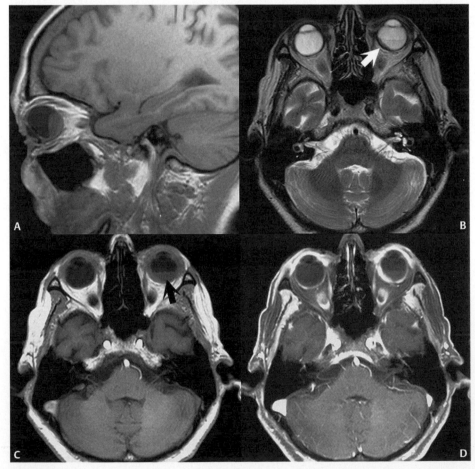

Figure 47–1

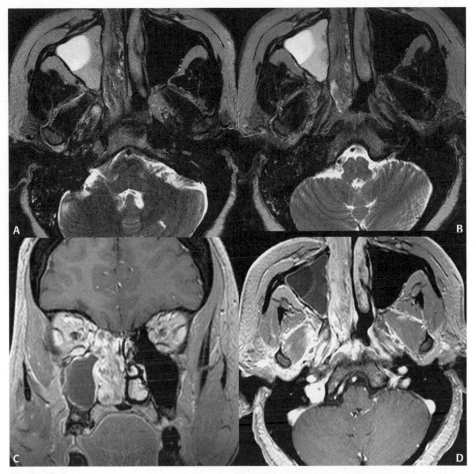

Figure 47–2

The retinal detachment is best seen on T1-weighted images posteriorly within the globe with intermediate signal intensity (black arrow). The metastasis itself is seen along the posterior medial wall of the globe with decreased signal intensity on the T2-weighted scan (white arrow) and focal abnormal contrast enhancement.

Scans from a patient with an inverted papilloma are presented in **Fig. 47–2**. A mass is noted within the right nasal cavity (middle meatus), with extension into the nasopharynx posteriorly and ethmoid sinus superiorly, causing obstruction of the right maxillary sinus—all classical imaging findings for this diagnosis. The upper half of **Fig. 47–2** features a comparison of field strength, with T2-weighted 3-mm sections at **(A)** 1.5 and **(B)** 3 T. These two scans were matched in terms of imaging technique (identical TR, TE, voxel size, bandwidth, and echo train), with the exception that **(B)** was acquired using a parallel imaging factor of two, resulting in a reduction of scan time from 2:48 to 1:36 min:sec. The pixel dimensions were 0.4 × 0.4 mm². The 1.5 and 3 T scans are equivalent diagnostically, with the 3 T scan substantially shorter with regard to acquisition time. Postcontrast **(C)** coronal and **(D)** axial T1-weighted scans at 3 T are also presented, acquired using the short TE GRE scan

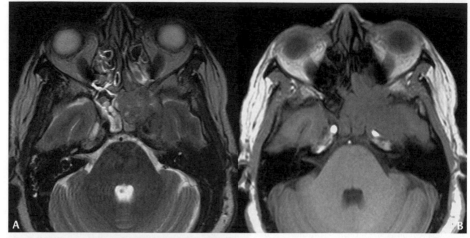

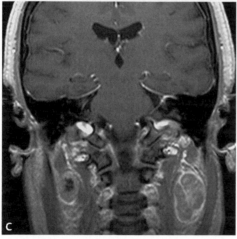

technique. These scans were 2 mm in slice thickness, with an acquisition time of 3:15 min:sec for each.

In **Fig. 47–3**, a destructive mass lesion is noted on axial **(A)** T2- and **(B)** T1-weighted images, with its epicenter in the left sphenoid sinus, extending into the nasal cavity and middle cranial fossa. Enlarged enhancing lymph nodes are noted on **(C)** the postcontrast coronal T1-weighted image, deep to the sternocleidomastoid muscles. Biopsy revealed squamous cell carcinoma. The slice thickness was 3 mm in each instance, with scan times of 1:05 to 1:22.

Figure 47–3

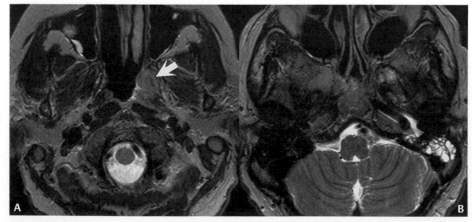

Figure 47–4

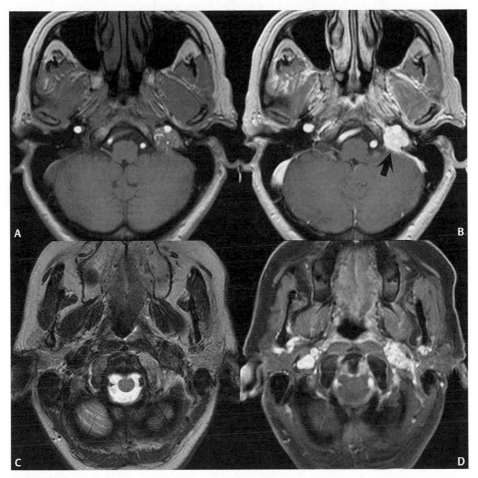

Figure 47-5

Figure 47-4 presents T2-weighted 3-mm images, acquisition time of 1:42, at two levels from a screening brain exam performed in a 52-year-old man with chronic headaches (left occipital in location). Abnormal soft tissue (arrow) obliterates the opening of the eustachian tube, thus causing an effusion in the left middle ear and mastoid sinus, and causes mass effect upon the fossa of Rosenmüller. Biopsy revealed grade 3, invasive squamous cell carcinoma. The tumor itself was seen on multiple adjacent 3-mm sections, illustrating the power of routine thin-section imaging.

Figure 47-5 presents axial **(A)** pre- and **(B)** postcontrast T1-, **(C)** T2-, and **(D)** postcontrast fat-saturated T1-weighted images of a 63-year-old woman with a glomus jugulare paraganglioma: **(A, B)** are at the level of the jugular bulb and **(C, D)** are more caudal. A hypervascular mass is noted (arrow), centered at the jugular foramen, with caudal intraluminal jugular vein extension. The lesion has a characteristic "salt and pepper" appearance, with small foci of high signal intensity precontrast on the T1-weighted image and low signal intensity on the T2-weighted image, due to flow phenomena. The slice thickness was 3 mm, with scan times of 1:11 to 1:56.

Brain: Pediatric Imaging

Robert A. Zimmerman and Val M. Runge

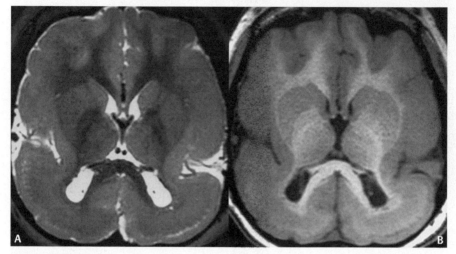

Figure 48–1

Given the improved SNR compared with 1.5 T, 3 T MR imaging holds particular promise for pediatric brain imaging. High-resolution 3D imaging is feasible, with realistic acquisition times (<5 min) for voxel sizes of 1 mm³ and under, with both T1- and T2-weighted scans possible (as well as FLAIR). Three-dimensional scans of the brain are typically acquired in either the sagittal or the axial orientation, with images subsequently reformatted in any additional desired plane. Complex anomalies are in particular well studied by high-resolution 3D imaging. The MR image of a 7-year-old patient with intractable seizures due to lissencephaly, a neuronal migration abnormality, is illustrated in **Fig. 48–1** with axial **(A)** T2- and **(B)** T1-weighted scans. The slice thicknesses for these 3D acquisitions, acquired in an axial orientation, were 1.5 and 0.9 mm, respectively.

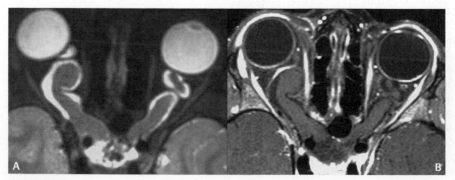

Figure 48–2

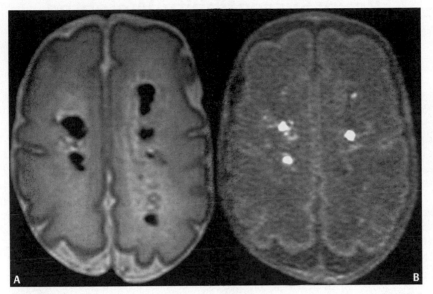

Figure 48–3

T2- and T1-weighted axial images, in a patient with neurofibromatosis type 1 (NF1) and bilateral optic nerve gliomas, are illustrated in **Figs. 48–2A** and **48–2B**. There is fusiform enlargement of the optic nerves bilaterally. The T2-weighted scan was acquired using 3D technique, with a slice thickness of 0.8 mm, and the postcontrast T1-weighted scan was acquired with 2D technique, and a slice thickness of 2 mm.

Axial T2-and T1-weighted images are illustrated in **Figs. 48–3A and 48–3B** from the exam of a 28-week premature, 2-week-old infant. Parenchymal hemorrhages are noted bilaterally. Both scans were 3D in type, with the images illustrated 1.5 and 0.9 mm in thickness, respectively, and the T1-weighted scan reconstructed from a sagittal primary acquisition.

The improved depiction of intracranial vessels at 3 T, using 3D TOF MRA, offers a further important advance for pediatric neuroimaging. Illustrated in **Figs. 48–4A and 48–4B** are 3D TOF MRA studies at 1.5 and 3 T in an 8-year-old sickle cell patient, with multiple prior strokes now presenting with transient ischemic attacks. The left internal carotid artery is not visualized on the 1.5 T study, other than the carotid terminus. The small thread of the residual patent vessel is well seen on the 3 T exam (arrows, **B**).

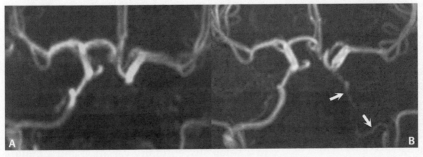

Figure 48–4

49 Brain: Susceptibility-Weighted Imaging

Stuart H. Schmeets

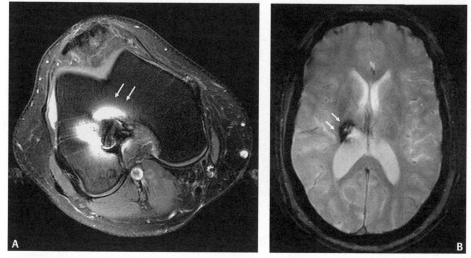

Figure 49–1

Magnetic susceptibility is defined as the degree to which a material will become magnetized when it is placed in the vicinity of a magnetic field. Two categories of magnetic susceptibility associated with MR imaging, ferromagnetism and paramagnetism, are demonstrated in **Fig. 49–1A** where a titanium screw has been placed to stabilize a popliteal anterior cruciate ligament (ACL) graft and **Fig. 49–1B** where high concentrations of iron in a chronic hemorrhage (arrows) are visualized with GRE acquisitions (arrows).

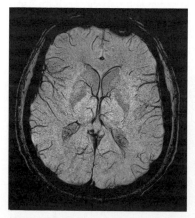

Figure 49–2

In each of the described examples, a material within the body exhibited the effects of magnetic susceptibility to a different degree than the tissues in its vicinity, resulting in a localized change in the magnetic field homogeneity. In **Fig. 49–1A**, the change in homogeneity was high and because magnetic field gradients are used to encode spatial information, this change in homogeneity produced distortions and variations in signal due to a significant shift in the resonant frequencies of protons in the region (arrows). In **Fig. 49–1B**, the magnetic susceptibility in the area of the lesion is only slightly higher than that in the rest of the brain, leading to a small susceptibility variation and a minute

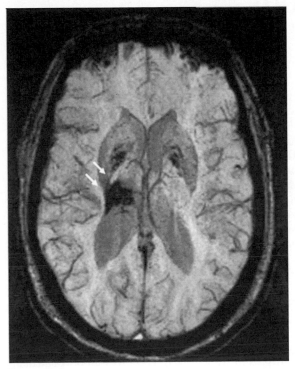

Figure 49–3

decrease in the SNR in the area of the lesion over adjacent tissues.

Because the effects of magnetic susceptibility double when the field strength is doubled, susceptibility effects can be exploited at higher magnetic fields to improve the diagnostic value of certain MR imaging techniques. One such technique generically termed *susceptibility-weighted imaging* (SWI) incorporates phase and/or magnitude reconstructions of a 3D GRE acquisition with an increased echo time designed to amplify the effect of magnetic susceptibility in the microvasculature of brain tissues. The 3D data set is thinly partitioned and a minimum intensity projection (minIP) of the data is processed to increase the delineation of small vessels as demonstrated in **Fig. 49–2**. This technique has shown clinical promise in augmenting the conspicuity of small infarcts (arrows) and delineation of the vascular pathways associated with abnormal tissues as shown in **Fig. 49–3**.

Susceptibility artifacts can negatively impact image quality at higher field strengths if not compensated for in routine imaging. **Figure 49–4** depicts a diffusion-weighted image where susceptibility artifacts have caused a distortion of tissues (arrows) in the frontal lobe of the brain. Currently, solutions such as parallel imaging minimize the effect these artifacts have on image quality. In the next few sections, we will discuss more susceptibility-based imaging techniques and how the higher field strength of 3 T MR imaging systems can be used to increase their clinical value.

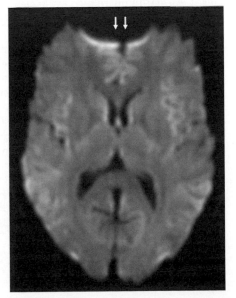

Figure 49–4

50 Brain: BOLD

Stuart H. Schmeets

The morphologic or structural information obtained during a routine MR imaging examination can be beneficial in the process of spatially localizing and diagnosing lesions within the brain. 3 T MR imaging systems provide additional SNR for faster acquisitions and/or higher spatial resolution. However, the process of presurgical planning requires a clear definition of the anatomic relationship between pathologic regions planned for resection and the relevant functional regions of the motor cortex that may be affected during the surgical procedure. This information cannot always be resolved from routine, T1- and T2-weighted MR imaging data sets, and because anatomic landmarks routinely used during surgical navigation may become distorted by tumor mass effect, noninvasive methods of mapping the motor cortex such as functional MR imaging can be incorporated to provide critical planning information to the neurosurgeon.

Functional MR imaging (fMRI), also called blood oxygen level dependent (BOLD) imaging, is a technique that benefits significantly from the increased effect of magnetic susceptibility on tissues examined at 3 T over 1.5 T systems. During fMRI procedures, the patient is asked to perform sequential tasks (termed *paradigms*), such as finger tapping, which induce an increase in oxygen consumption within the regions of the cortex associated with the task and signal surrounding vessels to begin to supply the area with a surplus of oxygen-rich blood to support continued activity. **Figure 50–1** demonstrates a diagram of some of the regions of interest of the motor cortex.

The exposed iron found in the molecular structure of deoxygenated hemoglobin causes normal brain tissues to display an intrinsic level of magnetic susceptibility based on the ratio of oxygenated to deoxygenated blood within the vasculature. The increase in oxygenated blood supplied to activated regions of the motor cortex changes these levels and leads to a small increase in the signal due to the reduction in localized magnetic susceptibility **(Fig. 50–2)**.

Figures 50–3A and **50–3B** demonstrate an fMRI examination performed on 1.5 T and 3 T MR imaging systems, respectively. During this finger-tapping experiment, the patient was asked to alternate between right- and left-sided activity leading to the visualization of bilateral activation. The increase in the effect of magnetic susceptibility between adjacent tissues with varied levels of deoxyhemoglobin causes a higher susceptibility variation between activated and nonactivated regions in the

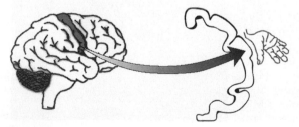

Figure 50–1

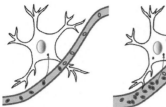

• = Oxygenated blood
○ = Deoxygenated blood

Figure 50–2

3 T experiment, resulting in a greater BOLD response and clearer delineation of activated borders. An additional important observation is the ipsilateral activation associated with the task that is visualized in the cerebellum to a limited extent at 1.5 T but quite pronounced at 3 T in this example, **Figs. 50–3C** and **50–3D**.

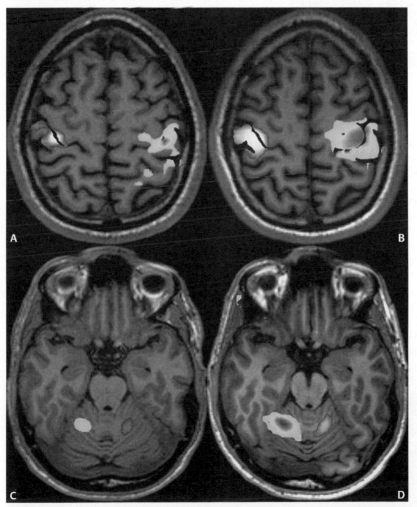

Figure 50–3

51 Brain: Perfusion

Stuart H. Schmeets

Figure 51-1

Cerebral MR perfusion imaging is a minimally invasive technique designed to assess differences in the hemodynamic properties of blood flow to the vascular bed of the brain by way of signal changes induced due to the rapid administration of a contrast agent during data acquisition. The increase in the effect of the magnetic susceptibility of tissues examined on 3 T MR systems is once again used to improve the image quality of this technique.

When MR pulse sequences that are highly sensitive to magnetic susceptibility differences are acquired during contrast administration, the paramagnetic characteristics of the MR contrast agent cause an overall reduction in SNR by increasing the susceptibility variation between areas of high and low concentration (e.g., vessels and brain tissues). This leads to an increase in localized proton dephasing, thus providing the basis for cerebral MR perfusion imaging. The first and most common method of perfusion imaging involves the bolus administration of a gadolinium chelate while specialized echoplanar pulse sequences are rapidly acquired covering the brain every 1.5 sec, providing the clinician the ability to plot changes in susceptibility (and thus blood flow) during the wash-in and wash-out phases of the injected contrast.

The degree of gadolinium-induced signal change during the acquisition is vitally important in image evaluation and is assessed by the calculation of a global bolus plot as shown in **Fig. 51-1**. The global bolus plot corresponds to the signal-intensity changes visible in the images shown in **Fig. 51-2**, which were extracted from the full data set at specific time points.

Several images or "maps" are generated based on the variations in the temporal rate of signal-to-noise change during the image acquisition. These variances in rate can be traced to an increase or decrease in blood flow or volume to a region of tissue. **Figure 51-3A** depicts a time-to-peak map in which regions of brain tissue demonstrating higher signal intensity represent regions where the arrival of contrast was

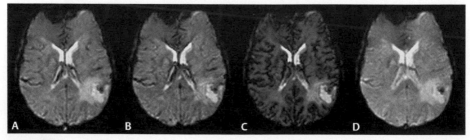

Figure 51-2

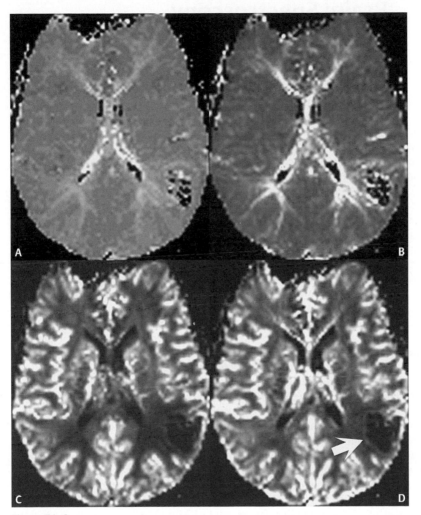

Figure 51–3

delayed compared with the rest of the brain. The percent-baseline-peak map depicted in **Fig. 51–3B** demonstrates the percentage of baseline signal that remains at the peak of the contrast bolus. Because the peak of the contrast bolus should represent the lowest SNR, regions displaying a greater percentage of the baseline signal, or brighter intensity are likely to be perfusing at a slower rate. **Figures 51–3C** and **51–3D** depict relative cerebral blood volume (CBV) and relative cerebral blood flow (CBF) maps in this patient with a large necrotic metastasis. The edema peripheral to the lesion demonstrates low CBV and CBF, while the thin rim of metabolically active tumor demonstrates increased CBV and CBF (arrow)—which surrounds the large central necrotic center.

Cerebral perfusion is commonly incorporated as an adjunct to DWI to assess cerebral ischemia but can also be applied to differentiate radiation-induced necrosis from recurrent tumor or simply to assess the overall degree of vascularity in the area of abnormal tissue or a suspected lesion.

52 Brain: Spectroscopy

Stuart H. Schmeets

Knowledge of the chemical composition of tissue samples can be especially useful in classifying and specifying abnormalities within the body. Radiologic conclusions obtained during routine imaging procedures are often confirmed with biopsies or microscopic analysis after resection. Magnetic resonance spectroscopy offers the clinician the ability to quantitatively analyze the chemical environment of tissues noninvasively, leading to an improvement in diagnostic accuracy and reducing patient discomfort.

Magnetic resonance spectroscopy (MRS) information of important metabolic markers is derived from the differences in the nuclear magnetic resonance frequency of nuclei within an externally applied magnetic field. Although the external field remains the same, angular frequency variations occur when a nucleus is shielded from the external field by other nuclei or electrons within its environment. Therefore, the resulting spectrum of frequencies is derived from the various degrees of shielding within the volume.

Increasing the strength of the external magnetic field to 3 T provides several benefits in MRS. As discussed in earlier chapters, the number of nuclei aligning in parallel to the external field, and thus providing signal, increases improving the SNR of NMR experiments and providing for the detection of metabolites whose quantities are normally too small to be seen at 1.5 T as well as providing a more accurate overall quantification of metabolite ratios. The added SNR can be employed to improve spectroscopic results in two additional ways. First, because MRS experiments normally require long acquisition times, the possibility of patient motion is of significant concern. A higher SNR allows the clinician to acquire spectroscopic information of a given volume of interest at 3 T in half the time of a 1.5 T experiment. **Figures 52–1A** and **52–1B** depict a 1H spectrum acquired on the same subject at both 1.5 T and 3 T, respectively. In the 3 T experiment, the number of signal averages and thus the acquisition time was reduced by a factor of two.

Second, spectroscopic experiments provide information that is averaged over the entire volume of interest. An increase in SNR allows the clinician to reduce the size of the volume examined to improve the specificity of the procedure yet maintain an acceptable level of signal, providing for example a significant advantage in regions such as the myocardium.

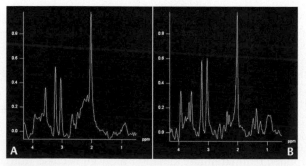

Figure 52–1

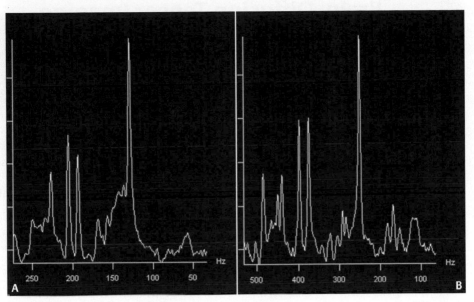

Figure 52–2

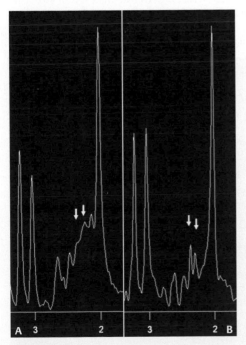

Figure 52–3

Another benefit of increasing the external field strength is that the change due to variations in the shielding of nuclei increases resulting in a greater frequency separation or chemical shift of metabolite peaks. **Figures 52–2A** and **52–2B** illustrate how an increase in the field strength from 1.5 T **(A)** to 3 T **(B)** results in a linear increase in resonant frequencies. This means that at 1.5 T, the 1H spectroscopy range covers ~300 Hz, but at 3 T the range is extended to ~600 Hz.

This becomes especially important when attempting to resolve metabolites with relatively small variations in frequency, as is the case with the glutamine and glutamate (GLX) groups. **Figures 52–3A** and **52–3B** demonstrate how the GLX frequencies overlap and are difficult to resolve at 1.5 T **(A)** but are more clearly defined at 3 T **(B)** (arrows). Although obstacles such as susceptibility effects and RF penetration can diminish the quality of the data, 3 T systems provide a clear advantage in MR spectroscopy.

53 Brain: Diffusion Tensor Imaging

Stuart H. Schmeets

The Brownian motion of water molecules within the brain has, for many years, been imaged with a specialized MR technique termed *diffusion-weighted imaging* (DWI) (see Case 29). This technique often incorporates information about diffusion in the slice, read, and phase direction, which limits the amount of magnitude and directional information that can be extracted. Diffusion tensor imaging (DTI) builds on the DWI technique to provide greater details of the directional component of the diffusion-based motion resulting in a diffusion analysis from which information on the microscopic structure of white-matter tracts can be inferred.

Once again, 3 T MR imaging systems prove superior to 1.5 T systems by providing higher SNR and improving the clinician's ability to quantify diffusion motion and direction. This SNR improvement is demonstrated in a normal volunteer in **Figs. 53–1A** and **53–1B** where data from a single diffusion slice with a b-value of 1000 s·mm^2 is illustrated at 1.5 T and 3 T, respectively.

Calculating the tensor of all 12 diffusion directions in the above experiment makes it possible to process a variety of images related to the magnitude and direction of molecular diffusion. **Figures 53–2A** and **53–2B** demonstrate the magnitude data of the diffusion tensor from the above experiment due to anisotropy. This image, termed a *fractional anisotropy* (FA) image, displays the magnitude of diffusion on a voxel by voxel basis. Although similar, the 3 T **(B)** image provides a better delineation of structural borders, for example the external capsule (arrow, **B**), due to increased SNR.

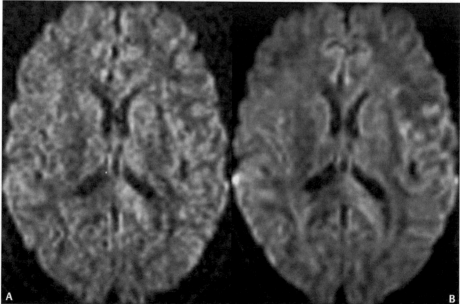

Figure 53–1

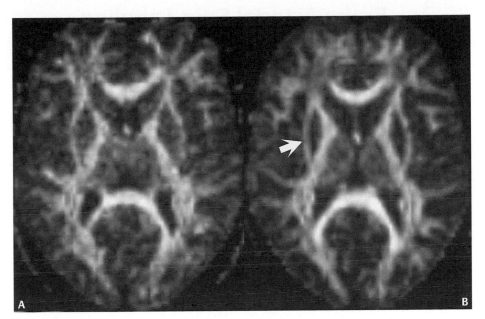

Figure 53–2

Within white matter tracts, diffusion is impeded perpendicular to the long axis of the fibers. Because DTI provides directional information within each voxel, the structure of white-matter tracts can also be calculated and reconstructed from the diffusion data. The images in **Figs. 53–3A** and **53–3B** are reconstructed from the data sets illustrated in **Fig. 53–2**. However, in these images the white-matter tracts have been calculated starting at the level of the medulla and reconstructing in the caudal to cranial direction. Note once again that the improvement in SNR plays a role in providing additional information at 3 T, regarding existence of crossing tracts (arrow, **B**), that can only be visualized in a limited way at 1.5 T (**A**).

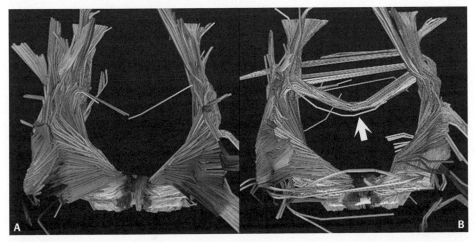

Figure 53–3

54 Brain: Arterial Spin-Labeling

Ronald L. Wolf

Clinical perfusion techniques use tracers in two basic categories: *diffusible* (the tracer is not confined to the vessels and enters the tissue) and *nondiffusible* (the tracer is confined to the vessels). Arterial spin-labeled (ASL) perfusion MR imaging is an example of a diffusible tracer technique. Arterial blood water is labeled and allowed to flow into the imaging plane(s), during which time there is T1 decay of the label. Multiple labeled/control image pairs are acquired and averaged. Subtraction of labeled images from unlabeled control images yields a difference image, in which the signal change is proportional to cerebral blood flow (CBF). Implementations include *pulsed* (PASL) or *continuous* (CASL) labeling methods. Nondiffusible MR perfusion techniques (dynamic susceptibility contrast, or DSC) involve analysis of the transient decrease in signal intensity on T2*-weighted images, observed during the first pass of contrast after intravenous bolus gadolinium chelate administration.

Figure 54–1 shows CBF maps of a glioblastoma (arrow) using **(A)** DSC and **(B)** CASL perfusion MR methods at 1.5 T and 3 T, respectively. A limitation of ASL methods compared with DSC perfusion MR methods is low SNR. Signal changes in gray matter for DSC perfusion MR imaging are of the order 20% for SE echoplanar imaging (EPI) and greater than 25% for GRE EPI (even more if the contrast dose is increased), while signal changes are of the order 1% or less for ASL at 1.5 T. Increased field strength provides an approximately twofold increase in SNR at 3 T compared with 1.5 T. Resolution for CASL is lower here (matrix 64 × 64 versus 128 × 128 for

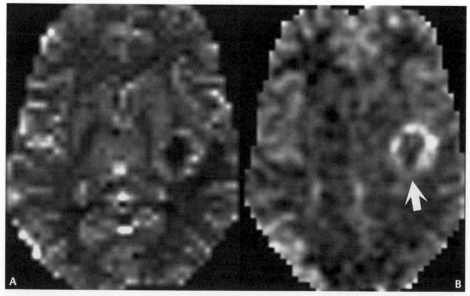

Figure 54–1

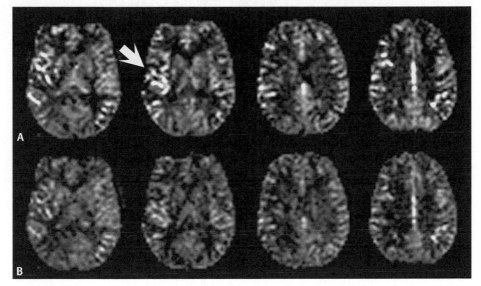

Figure 54–2

DSC), but image quality is comparable with less large vessel signal and also a relative insensitivity to permeability.

Another benefit of higher field strength is improved labeling efficiency due to increased T1. With ASL methods, transit delays resulting from cervicocranial stenotic-occlusive disease may cause artifacts such as persistent label in large vessels. Selected CASL perfusion MR images from a patient with moyamoya disease are shown in **Fig. 54–2**. Two acquisitions were acquired at 3 T, with delay times between labeling and measurement of **(A)** 1500 msec and **(B)** 1800 msec. These demonstrate right greater than left bright signal in large vessels, especially in the right middle cerebral artery territory (arrow) at a delay time of 1500 msec **(A)**. The large vessel signal represents labeled spins experiencing enough of a delay that exchange with the microvasculature or tissue has not yet occurred. At 1800 msec **(B)**, most of the intravascular signal has passed into the microvasculature and tissue. One can also appreciate that the SNR has decreased slightly as the label is decaying with time constant T1. The long delay times shown here are problematic at 1.5 T but made possible at 3 T due to the inherent greater SNR.

There are additional ways of increasing SNR in ASL studies. For example, use of CASL yields another ~30% gain in SNR compared with the PASL method. Other sources of potential improvement in SNR include improved background suppression, use of pseudo continuous labeling for improved labeling efficiency, use of single-shot 3D gradient and spin echo (GRASE) sequences, implementation of parallel imaging, and improvements in coil technology.

55 Spine: Cervical—Introduction

Val M. Runge and William H. Faulkner Jr.

As with imaging in the head, there is a substantial improvement in SNR with current cervical spine coil designs at 3 T when compared with 1.5 T. This has yet to be quantified and may vary among manufacturers. Given the gain in SNR, the dilemma is faced, as in the brain, whether to use this increase to shorten scan time or to improve spatial resolution. Probably the greatest limitation in cervical spine imaging at 1.5 T is slice thickness, given the small structures involved—the disk space, cord, and neural foramina. In our experience, the decision is clear—that the improved SNR at 3 T should be used to decrease slice thickness.

Illustrated in **Fig. 55–1** are sagittal FSE T2-weighted images at 1.5 T in a 73-year-old patient with a history of surgical fusion of C5–6 in the distant past. Broad diskosteophyte complexes are noted at the interspace above and below the fusion, due to accentuated motion at these levels. The images were acquired in 3:12 min:sec, with a slice thickness of 4 mm and a 25% interslice gap. Due to the slice thickness, the cervical cord is really only imaged on the single central slice, with partial volume imaging of the edges of the cord on the two slices just off the midline.

This depiction of the cord at 1.5 T differs substantially from that seen in **Fig. 55–2** at 3 T, when a 2-mm slice thickness is used (the interslice gap was 10%). Scan time was 2:28 min:sec, slightly shorter than the 1.5 T exam, with in-plane resolution (pixel dimensions) approximated to be that of the 1.5 T exam. At 3 T (**Fig. 55–2**), using 2-mm sections, portions of the cord are seen on six slices, as opposed to three at 1.5 T. The degree of canal stenosis secondary to the disk osteophyte complexes present at C4–5

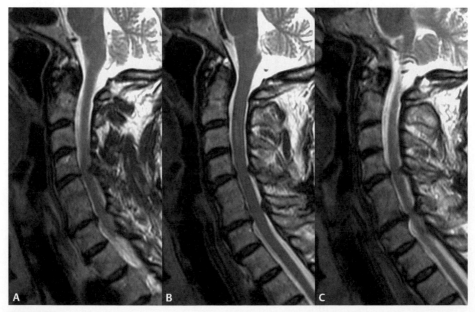

Figure 55–1

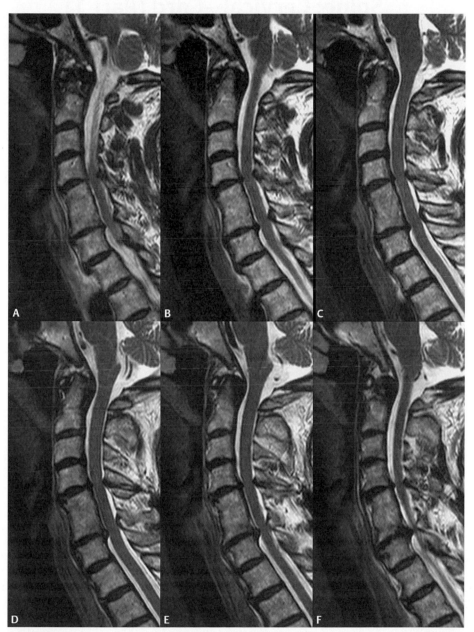

Figure 55–2

and C6–7 is better depicted. Not illustrated, but clearly evident from clinical experience, is the improvement in readability of the off midline sagittal images using a 2-mm slice thickness. Facet joint disease, whether an osteophyte or disk herniation extends later-ally, and even neural foraminal narrowing (despite their oblique course through the plane of section) are all substantially better depicted on thin-section imaging at 3 T.

56 Spine: Cervical—Cord (Part 1)
Val M. Runge

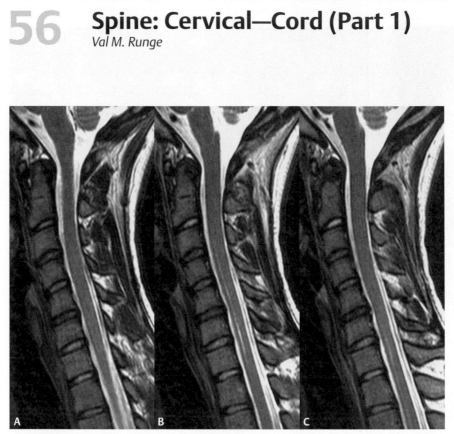

Figure 56–1

Cervical spine imaging at 3 T makes feasible routine 2-mm imaging, markedly improving visualization of cord abnormalities. **Figure 56–1** presents midline images from a 2:28 min:sec FSE T2-weighted scan, using a slice thickness of 2 mm with a 20% gap. The cord is visualized on all three images, with the middle image depicting mild dilatation of the

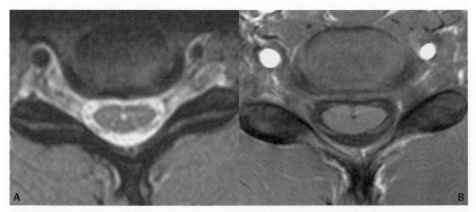

Figure 56–2

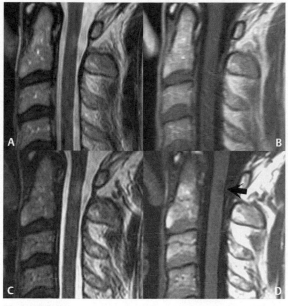

Figure 56–3

central canal (hydromyelia) extending from C4 to C7. This abnormality would likely have not been depicted at 1.5 T on sagittal scans, due to partial volume effects.

Dilatation of the central canal is confirmed on axial imaging (**Fig. 56–2**) with (**A**) 2D T2-weighted and (**B**) 3D T1-weighted GRE techniques. Note also the excellent depiction of cervical nerves, within the thecal sac, on both images.

The scans in **Figs. 56–3** and **56–4** are of a 54-year-old woman with an 8-year history of multiple sclerosis. Sagittal imaging at (A, B) 1.5 T and (**C, D**) 3 T using (A, C) T2- and (**B, D**) T1-weighted techniques are compared in **Fig. 56–3**. The slice thickness was 4 mm at 1.5 T and (**C**) 2 and (**D**) 3 mm at 3 T. Scan times were comparable, with (**A**), (**B**), and (**D**) each requiring ~3.5 min, with the exception that (**C**) the sagittal T2-weighted FSE scan at 3 T was shorter by 1 min. The large MS plaque at C1–2 is equally well demonstrated at 1.5 and 3 T on T2-weighted scans, despite the reduction in slice thickness at 3 T. On T1-weighted imaging, the lesion is only visualized at 3 T, due to the improved tissue contrast of the T1-FLAIR technique, with subtle cord atrophy also noted (arrow). On axial imaging (**Fig. 56–4**), T2-weighted GRE images of the lower cervical cord acquired at (**A**) 1.5 T and (**B**) 3 T are compared. A small MS plaque is noted posteriorly within the cord, slightly to the left of midline, difficult to detect at 1.5 T but clearly visualized (due to reduced partial volume effects) at 3 T (arrow). Scan times were 5:10 and 4:24, with slice thicknesses of 4 and 2 mm, respectively, at 1.5 and 3 T.

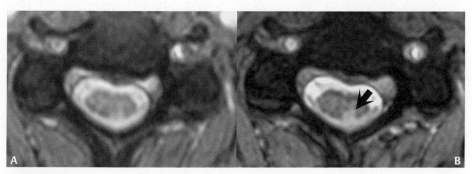

Figure 56–4

57 Spine: Cervical—Cord (Part 2)
Val M. Runge

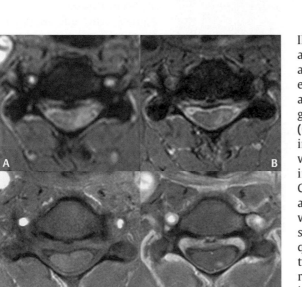

Figure 57–1

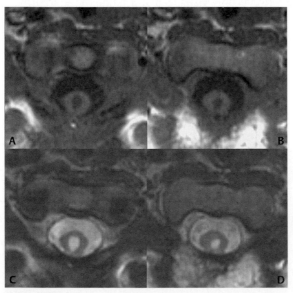

Figure 57–2

Illustrated in **Fig. 57–1** are axial T2-weighted GRE scans at **(A)** 1.5 and **(B)** 3 T, together with pre- and postcontrast axial T1-weighted spoiled gradient echo (VIBE) scans **(C, D)** at 3 T. For T1-weighted imaging of the cervical spine, we favor the use of 2D FLAIR in the sagittal plane (see Case 56) and 3D VIBE in the axial plane. The axial T2-weighted scan at 3 T is substantially improved in image quality when compared with that at 1.5 T, due in part to reduced partial volume imaging (4 versus 3 mm sections). The axial T1-weighted scan at 1.5 T (not shown) was similarly poor relative to its counterpart at 3 T. Within the cord, there is edema adjacent to a small enhancing lesion, likely inflammatory in nature.

Figure 57–2 presents 4-mm axial T1- and T2-weighted scans at 1.5 T in a patient several years after resection of an ependymoma, demonstrating a postoperative cavity. **Figures 57–3** and **57–4** present 3-mm postcontrast T1- and T2-weighted scans at 3 T in the same patient. The improved depiction of the postsurgical cavity (seen on four consecutive slices at 3 T as compared with two at 1.5 T) is due to the smaller section thickness, combined with the lack of a gap between slices (for both the 2D and 3D

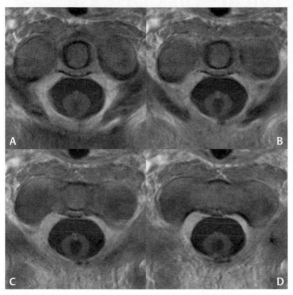

scans). Note the clear depiction of cervical nerves within the thecal sac, together with subtle enhancement within the cord anterior to the resection cavity and where scar tethers the cord posteriorly, features only seen at 3 T.

Figure 57–3

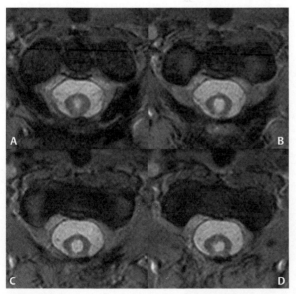

Figure 57–4

58 Spine: Cervical—Disk Disease

Val M. Runge

3 T provides a clinically important improvement, in terms of diagnostic image quality, for the evaluation of cervical disk disease. The slice thicknesses used in routine practice at 1.5 T are simply too large for reliable, consistent assessment of disk herniations and neural foraminal compromise, despite being currently accepted as the gold standard. 3 T offers the ability to obtain substantially thinner sections within a realistic scan time, diminishing markedly the problems due to partial volume imaging. Illustrated in **Fig. 58–1** are four adjacent sagittal T2-weighted sections from a SPACE acquisition at 3 T (the voxel dimensions for this 3D scan were $0.8 \times 0.8 \times 0.9$ mm^3). Shown are four near-midline images from this 72-slice acquisition. Note the excellent delineation of cord, CSF, and the disk/CSF interface. Of particular note is the uniform high signal intensity of CSF, without evidence of CSF pulsation artifacts. A moderate-sized central disk herniation is noted at C5–6 with some caudal extension of disk material posterior to the C6 vertebral body. SPACE provides for high-resolution reformatted images in any desired plane, all reconstructed from the single primary acquired data set, making possible markedly improved visualization of disk herniations in the axial plane as well, together with the possibility for assessment of the neural foramina in true cross section (double oblique).

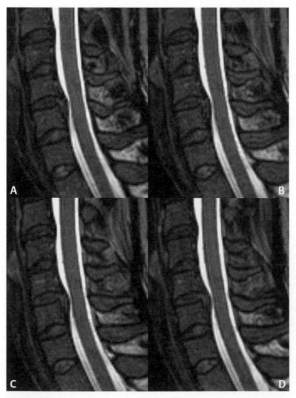

Illustrated in **Fig. 58–2** are four consecutive axial T2-weighted images through the disk herniation also shown in **Fig. 58–1**. The slice thickness was 2 mm (10% gap), with a scan time of 5:33. **Figure 58–3** presents the matching T1-weighted sections (2.2-mm thickness, no gap) acquired in 4:43 using 3D VIBE. There is excellent depiction of the disk herniation itself, due in part to visualization on multiple adjacent thin sections. **Figure 58–4** presents 16 consecutive images from the 6:02 min:sec SPACE exam illustrated with limited sections in **Fig. 58–1**, revealing graphically the effect of thin-section imaging.

Caveats do exist of course for 3 T imaging of the cervical

Figure 58–1

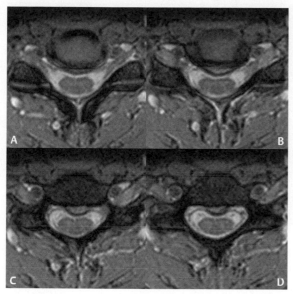

Figure 58–2

spine, with image degradation due to gross patient motion and CSF pulsation (the latter on 2D FSE scans) being two. The sagittal FSE T2-weighted scan **(Fig. 58–5A)** in this patient is nondiagnostic due to CSF pulsation artifacts, which are markedly improved by pulse gating **(Fig. 58–5B)**. This phenomenon is not however restricted

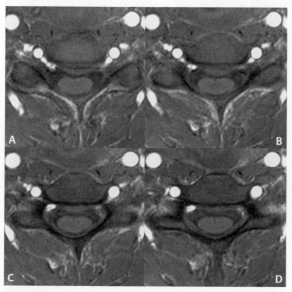

Figure 58–3

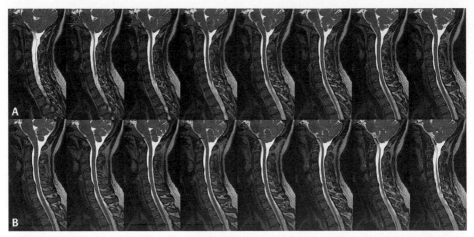

Figure 58–4

to 3 T, with the 1.5 T sagittal T2-weighted scan **(Fig. 58–6)** in this patient similarly degraded due to CSF pulsation artifacts. Scan time for the gated image presented in **Fig. 58–5B** was 2:04 min with a slice thickness of 2 mm.

Illustrated in **Fig. 58–7** is a comparison of axial scans in the same patient at **(A, B)** 1.5 and **(C, D)** 3 T. Scan times in this instance were all ~3.5 mins, whether for the T2-weighted 2D GRE **(A, C)**, the T1-weighted 2D SE (B), or the T1-weighted 3D VIBE **(D)**

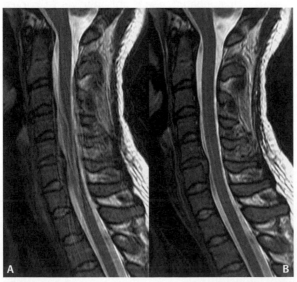

Figure 58–5

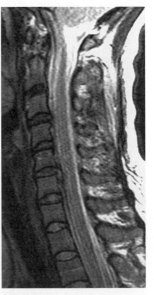

Figure 58–6

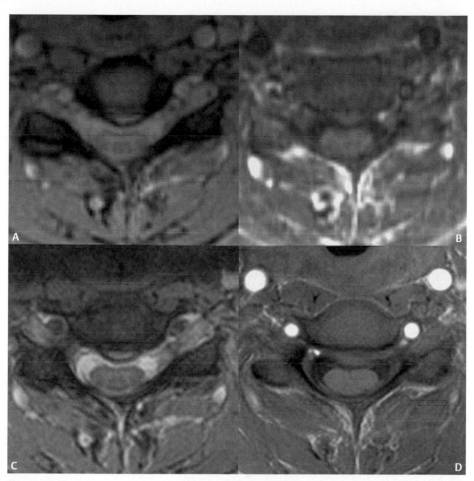

Figure 58–7

scan, regardless of field strength. The scans at 1.5 T have a lower in-plane resolution and are also thicker in section (4 mm with a 1-mm gap as opposed to 3 mm with no gap at 3 T in this instance). All scans had slice coverage from C2–3 through C7–T1, standard for our institution. Although radiologists have come to accept axial imaging at 1.5 T as the gold standard, the axial images at 3 T in this instance provide better delineation of the cord (and the mild contouring due to this disk herniation), the relevant cervical nerves (well seen on the axial T1-weighted exam), and the CSF–disk interface.

Illustrated in **Fig. 58–8** are 3-mm contiguous 2D T2-weighted GRE scans through a small chronic central disk herniation at C3–4 (note the small osteophyte above

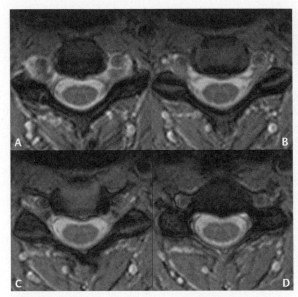

Figure 58–8

and below). **Figure 58–9** presents the 3-mm 3D T1-weighted VIBE images at the same levels. Scan times were 3:53 and 3:46, respectively. Note also the excellent visualization of the neural foramina at 3 T (seen on three consecutive images), made possible due to use of thin adjacent slices.

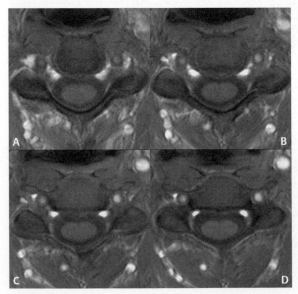

Figure 58–9

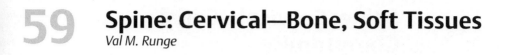

59 Spine: Cervical—Bone, Soft Tissues
Val M. Runge

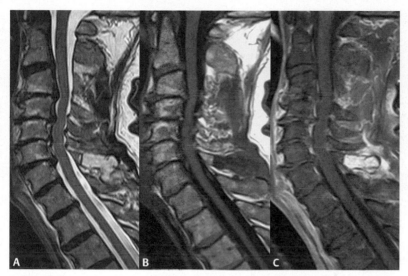

Figure 59–1

Depiction of bone and soft tissue lesions involving the cervical spine is improved at 3 T when compared with 1.5 T, primarily due to thinner sections and shorter scan times, both made possible by a substantial improvement in SNR, together with excellent fat suppression. Illustrated in **Figs. 59–1** and **59–2** are sagittal and axial scans from a patient with a solid aneurysmal bone cyst. The lesion, which is expansile and involves the C7 spinous process (with an associated soft tissue component), is hyperintense on T2-weighted scans and hypointense on precontrast T1-weighted scans, and demonstrates prominent enhancement postcontrast. Note the excellent fat suppression on the postcontrast sagittal T1 FLAIR and axial 3D VIBE scans. The slice thickness was 2 mm for the sagittal T2-weighted FSE scan **(A)** and 3 mm for remaining scans, which included sagittal T1-FLAIR **(B, C)**, and axial T2-weighted GRE **(A)** and T1-weighted VIBE **(B, C)**.

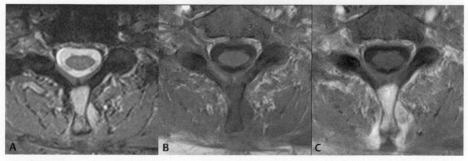

Figure 59–2

60 Spine: Cervical—Canal Compromise

Val M. Runge

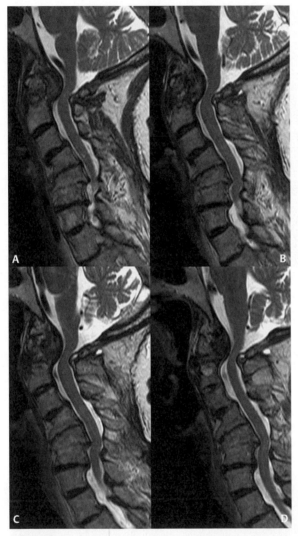

Figure 60–1

Figure 60-1 presents the four midline images from a T2-weighted FSE sagittal scan at 3 T in a patient with severe cervical spondylitic degenerative disease. The slice thickness was 2 mm with pixel dimensions of 1.0×0.6 mm^2. Although the degenerative changes at C4–6 are extensive, the patient presents with mild quadriparesis and loss of fine motor control in both hands, findings referable to the lesion at C1–2. At this level, there is moderate cord flattening and moderate to severe central canal stenosis, due to compression both anteriorly and posteriorly, the former by abundant soft tissue which erodes the dens. The availability of thin-section imaging at 3 T, in both the sagittal (as illustrated) and axial planes, for the cervical spine markedly improves depiction of canal compromise and on this basis diagnostic efficacy.

61 Spine: Cervicothoracic Junction
Val M. Runge

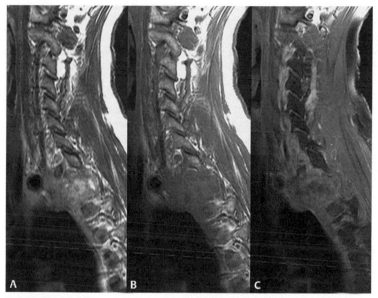

Figure 61–1

A major advance in recent years has been the implementation of integrated coils, allowing seamless imaging of adjacent anatomic areas. In the past, some anatomic regions, like the cervicothoracic junction, were poorly imaged simply because the area lay in a transition zone, covered poorly by the coil above (cervical) and that below (thoracic/lumbar). On modern systems, these regions no longer represent a challenge and are well imaged—whether at 1.5 or 3 T. Illustrated in **Figs. 61–1A** to **61–1C** is a Pancoast tumor on sagittal 3 T T2-, T1-, and postcontrast fat-suppressed T1-weighted images. On axial T1- and T2-weighted images at 3 T (**Figs. 61–2 A** and **61–2B**), vertebral body and rib invasion is well depicted, together with visualization of the apical lung mass itself. The slice thickness was 3 to 4 mm, with scan times (for one concatenation) of 1:36 to 2:36, with two concatenations required in each instance due to a combination of SAR limits and required number of slices.

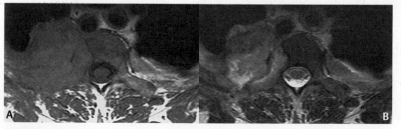

Figure 61–2

62 Spine: Thoracic—Introduction

Val M. Runge

Thoracic spine imaging has always represented a challenge for MR. Of the three major anatomic regions (cervical, thoracic, and lumbar), the thoracic spine has been the area least well imaged. Respiration and cardiac motion are two major reasons. For imaging at 3 T, where all measures must be taken to limit image degradation due to motion artifacts, sagittal imaging should be performed with phase encoding in the cranial–caudal direction. Illustrated in **Fig. 62–1** are **(A)** sagittal FSE T2-weighted, **(B)** FSE T1-weighted (three echoes), and **(C)** T1-FLAIR images of the thoracic spine in a 70-year-old patient with essentially a normal exam (a very small disk osteophyte complex is noted at T7–8). Scan times were 5:12, 3:30, and 5:12 mins:sec respectively. Two concatenations were required in each instance, resulting in these relatively long scan times. The slice thickness was 4 mm, with an FOV of 290 mm and pixel dimensions approximating 1 mm². In limited experience, thoracic spine imaging at 3 T is comparable with regard to image quality to that at 1.5 T, when attention is paid to limiting motion artifacts. It should be noted, however, that 3 T is in its infancy. Future improvements in coil technology likely will lead to a further increase in SNR. For T1-weighted imaging at 3 T, the choice lies between SE (or FSE) technique and T1-FLAIR. The latter offers improved cord-CSF contrast on T1-weighted scans (as illustrated), which is often poor with SE (or FSE) technique at 3 T. However, T1-FLAIR requires a longer scan time and is more sensitive to motion artifacts.

Figure 62–2 presents images at **(A, D)** 1.5 T and **(B, C, E, F)** 3 T in a patient with non–small cell lung carcinoma metastatic to T6 and T7. The slice thickness was 4 mm, with no attempt made to reduce scan times at 3 T when compared with 1.5 T. The 1.5 T

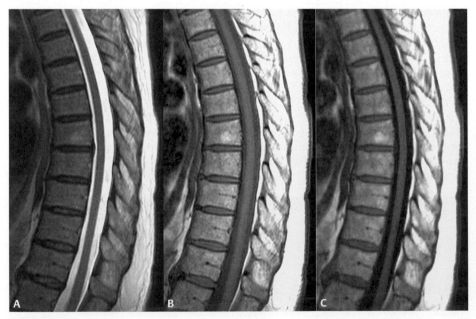

Figure 62–1

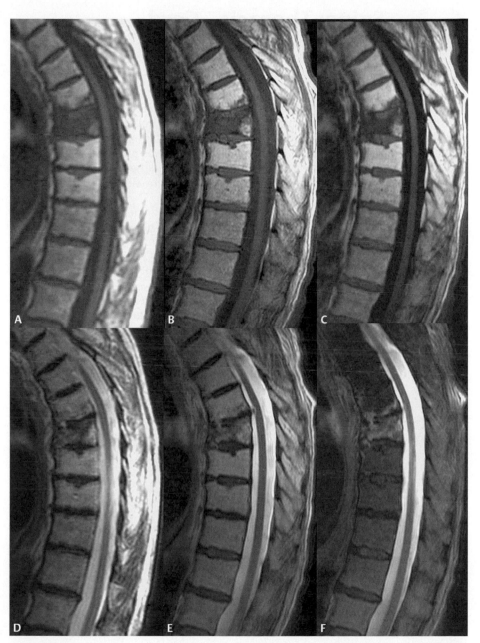

Figure 62–2

images are degraded to some extent due to the use of a larger pixel size. The near complete replacement of the T7 vertebral body with metastatic disease is well visualized on all T1-weighted scans, with (**C**) T1-FLAIR demonstrating slightly improved contrast between tumor and normal marrow, as well as between cord and CSF. Tumor involvement on T2-weighted scans is best depicted on the 3 T scan (**F**) with fat saturation.

63 Spine: Thoracic—Cord

Val M. Runge

Illustrated in **Fig. 63–1** are **(A, B)** T2-weighted FSE and **(C, D)** T1-weighted FLAIR sagittal images of the thoracic spine in a patient with hydromyelia of the lower thoracic cord. Acquisition times were 2:36 in each instance for one concatenation, with two concatenations required for both scans. The latter was principally for SAR reasons, showing the potential for reduced scan times even in the thoracic spine at 3 T—as compared with 1.5 T—when SAR reduction approaches such as VERSE are fully implemented.

In T1-weighted imaging of the cord at 3 T, studies have demonstrated that CNR (for spinal cord versus CSF) with T1 FLAIR is superior to T1 FSE, offering more than a threefold improvement. As a result, for imaging of the cord, T1 FLAIR is recommended. The inversion time with T1 FLAIR can be calculated to optimize CNR, with scan parameters of TR/TE/TI = 3500/12/1200 providing excellent cord-CSF contrast and to a first approximation an optimized scan.

Caveats abound in 3 T imaging of the thoracic spine. Attention should be paid to phase-encoding direction and proper placement of saturation pulses to minimize ghosting from the chest and heart. Long echo trains with FSE T2-weighted scans can lead to unacceptable blurring. However, artifacts from cerebrospinal fluid pulsation have not been as severe as anticipated and surprisingly do not appear to be more prominent than at 1.5 T.

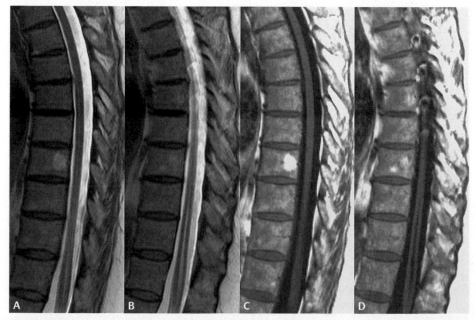

Figure 63–1

64 Spine: Lumbar—Disk Herniation (Part 1)

Benjamin Hyman and Val M. Runge

MR of the lumbar spine is the imaging modality of choice for the evaluation of disk disease, congenital malformations, infection, and neoplastic disease. Due to its higher SNR, 3 T holds the potential for improved diagnostic imaging of the lumbar spine, specifically with regard to either increased spatial resolution or decreased exam time. There are, however, still some challenges with 3 T before this can be fully realized. Issues due to the increased field strength, including specifically dielectric effect, SAR limitations, and motion/pulsation artifacts, are still being investigated in terms of optimizing 3 T for imaging of the lumbar spine. The improvements noted in 3 T imaging of the brain and cervical spine have not, to date, been fully realized in lumbar imaging, predominantly due to these limitations.

Figures 64–1A to **64–1D** illustrate this by comparison of T2-weighted images at 1.5 T (**A, C**) and 3 T (**B, D**) from a patient with a broad-based disk bulge at L4–L5 and a

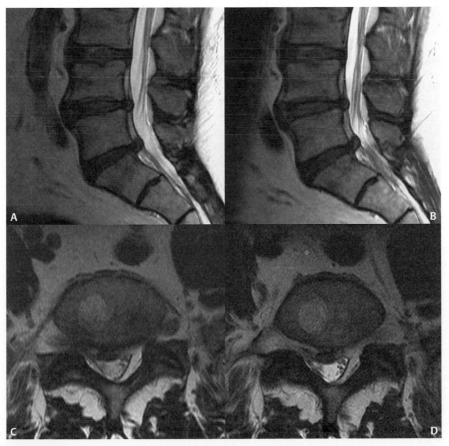

Figure 64–1

central/right paramedian disk herniation at L5–S1. Both the 1.5 T and 3 T images were obtained using a 4-mm slice thickness but differed (slightly) in time of acquisition (TA) and receiver bandwidth. At 1.5 T, the T2-weighted sagittal scan was acquired with the following parameters: TA = 4:08, bandwidth (BW) 130, and voxel size of 1.1 × 0.5 × 4.0 mm^3. Corresponding parameters for the remaining images included **(B)** 3 T with TA = 2:44 × 2, BW 255, 1.1 × 0.5 × 4 mm^3, **(C)** 1.5 T with TA 3:36, BW 195, 0.8 × 0.5 × 4 mm^3, and **(D)** 3 T with TA = 1:56 × 2, BW 250, 0.6 × 0.5 × 4 mm^3. There is little difference in diagnostic image quality and time of acquisition between the studies at 1.5 and 3 T, in this instance principally due to SAR limitations. The scan times at 3 T were double what might have been otherwise achieved due to the use of two concatenations (each scan in essence was acquired twice). Two concatenations were needed in both the axial and sagittal 3 T exams, but for different reasons. On the 3 T sagittal exam, two concatenations were selected to permit the scan to be run with the chosen parameters (with one concatenation, SAR limits would have been exceeded). Scan times will improve at 3 T relative to 1.5 T in lumbar spine imaging once SAR reduction methods are fully implemented (which is currently underway), allowing for more slices to be acquired in a single scan. The additional concatenation on the axial study was due to the number of slices acquired on the 3 T exam (19 slices) versus that on the 1.5 T exam (10 slices) and thus could have been eliminated if a lower number of slices had been acquired. Also demonstrated is the need for adjustment in receiver bandwidth. At 3 T, there is a greater difference in resonance frequency of fat and water protons leading to increased chemical shift artifact, if all other factors are held constant. To offset this effect and achieve a similar degree of pixel (chemical) shift at 1.5 and 3 T, a higher receiver bandwidth must be used, at the expense of some SNR. Another concern in imaging of the lumbar spine at 3 T is the potential for image degradation due to motion and pulsation artifacts from anterior structures. These are increased in magnitude relative to 1.5 T, emphasizing the importance of appropriate placement of the saturation slab just anterior to the lumbar spine. Also advocated is the choice of craniocaudal phase encoding for sagittal and left to right for axial scans. With this choice, artifact from motion propagates principally over areas of the image that are of little concern when evaluating the lumbar spine.

65 Spine: Lumbar—Disk Herniation (Part 2)

Benjamin Hyman and Val M. Runge

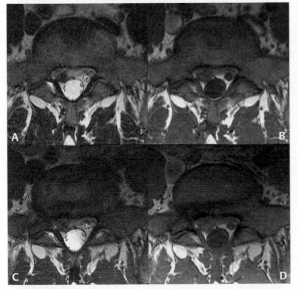

Figure 65–1

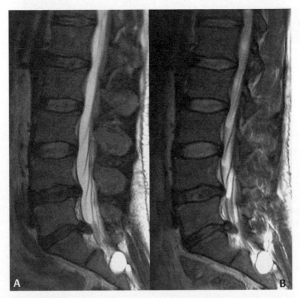

Figure 65–2

Figure 65–1 depicts a right paracentral disk herniation at L5–S1 that impinges upon the S1 nerve root just subsequent to its exit from the thecal sac: **(A, B)** are T2- (TA 4:55, voxel size of $0.8 \times 0.5 \times 4$ mm^3) and T1- (TA 2:45, $0.9 \times 0.6 \times 4$ mm^3) weighted images at 1.5 T; **(C, D)** are the corresponding T2- (TA 1:56, $0.6 \times 0.5 \times 4$ mm^3) and T1- (TA 2:42, $0.9 \times 0.6 \times 4$ mm^3) weighted images at 3 T. What is again seen, as in Case 64, is the relative equivalence of the depiction of pathology at the two field strengths. This is confirmed on the comparison of sagittal T2-weighted images **(Fig. 65–2)** from the same patient at **(A)** 1.5 and **(B)** 3 T. The equality of the images is largely related to SAR limitations at 3 T (at the time these images were acquired), with a subsequent software upgrade implementing several of the SAR reduction approaches currently under development. Yet, even without these advances, if one limits the extent of the exam to the level of disk pathology, the SAR limitations are bypassed, permitting acquisition of thin, high-resolution images with a scan time and quality not possible at 1.5 T.

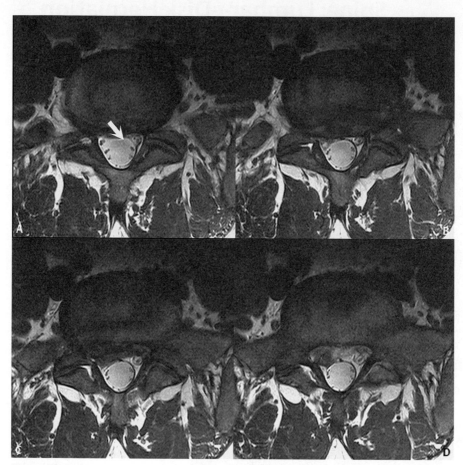

Figure 65–3

This approach is illustrated in **Fig. 65–3** on T2-weighted images (four adjacent slices are shown) acquired at 3 T (TA 4:28, voxel dimensions of $0.6 \times 0.5 \times 2.4$ mm^3). Due to the use of thin sections, depiction of the disk herniation and its impingement on S1 is improved. Thus a clear current advantage of 3 T over 1.5 T in the lumbar spine is the capability for thin-section imaging, revealing detail concerning nerve root compression. Incidentally seen in this image is an example of a dielectric effect (arrow), seen as a shading of CSF signal intensity from right to left within the thecal sac. This effect is more noticeable at 3 T secondary to increased B_1 field inhomogeneity, leading to signal attenuation. Further studies are in place to deal with RF field homogeneity, including the use of dielectric pads, optimization of RF transmitter coil arrangements, and normalization filters (see Case 8).

Figure 65–4 further demonstrates with T1-weighted axial images (eight contiguous slices are illustrated) at 3 T (TA = 4:31, 0.9 mm $\times$ 0.6 mm $\times$ 2 mm^3) the exquisite detail regarding the disk herniation and resultant nerve compression afforded by thin-section imaging. These 2-mm sections allow for close examination of an affected

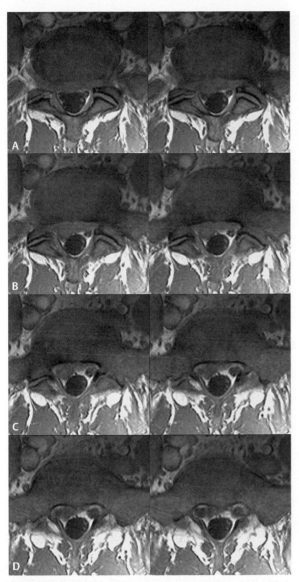

Figure 65–4

level not afforded by 1.5 T, which permits only slice thicknesses in the range of 3 to 4 mm (in a reasonable scan time). Thin-section imaging at higher field will provide the film reader with a combination of improved image quality, better structural detail, and increased ability to define and detect small lesions.

Figure 65–5 presents T2-weighted sagittal sections (four adjacent slices are illustrated) at 3 T using a 2.4-mm slice thickness (TA 5:58, $0.6 \times 0.5 \times 2.4$ mm^3), demonstrating the same disk herniation presented in **Fig. 65–2** but in much greater detail.

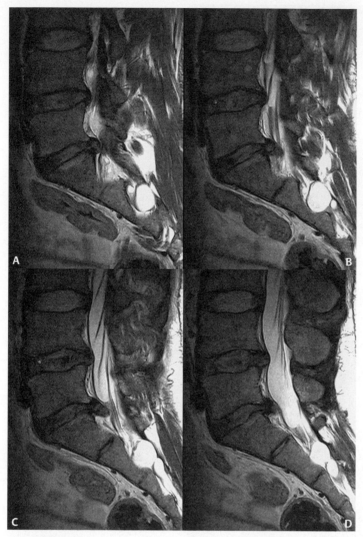

Figure 65–5

Characterization of the herniation and its relationship to adjacent nerves is possible from the multiple sections that detail the pathology, which is more difficult to do at 1.5 T. The best section width attained at 1.5 T was 4 mm, which allowed for visualization of the disk herniation itself on only a single slice.

66 Spine: Lumbar—Postoperative (Part 1)

Val M. Runge

1.5 T (**A**) and 3 T (**B**) lumbar spine images are compared in **Fig. 66–1**, **Fig. 66–2**, and **Fig. 66–3**. **Fig. 66–1** presents FSE T2-weighted sagittal scans, **Fig. 66–2** FSE T2-weighted axial scans (at L3–4), and **Fig. 66–3** FSE postcontrast T1-weighted axial scans (at L4–5). The two MR exams were acquired consecutively (the scans at 3 T were acquired first), with the patient being a 37-year-old man with a left laminotomy at L4–5 performed 6 years prior to the current exam. He now presents with right-sided pain in an L4 nerve root distribution.

The slice thickness was 4 mm in each instance. Scan times and voxel sizes were similar for all comparisons. Bandwidth was adjusted for equivalent pixel shift. The sagittal T2-weighted scans are comparable at 1.5 and 3 T in terms of diagnostic quality, demonstrating disk desiccation at L3–4 through L5–S1, and end-plate degenerative changes at L4–5. A right paracentral disk herniation at L3–4 is noted on both sagittal and axial T2-weighted scans and is equally well depicted at 1.5 and 3 T. On the axial scans (**Fig. 66–2**), the right L4 nerve is noted to be compressed in the lateral recess by the disk herniation. A reduced flip angle (120 degrees in the axial plane and 135 degrees in the sagittal plane, for refocusing) was employed for SAR reasons at 3 T.

Figure 66–3 presents axial T1-weighted images at L4–5 after IV gadolinium chelate administration at (**A**) 1.5 and (**B**) 3 T. The 1.5 T scan was performed in a delayed fashion

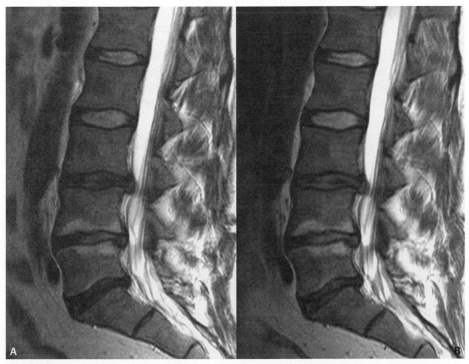

Figure 66–1

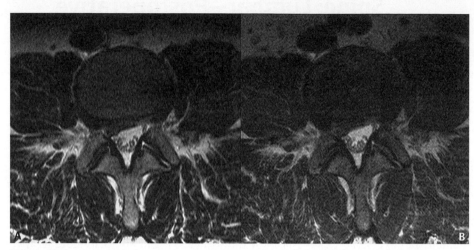

Figure 66–2

after contrast administration, accounting for the decreased enhancement of scar noted on that exam (relative to the exam at 3 T). The left-sided laminotomy, mild postoperative deformity of the thecal sac, and enhancing scar tissue surrounding the exiting L5 nerve root (arrow) on the left are all well visualized on (B) the 3 T exam. Both the 1.5 and 3 T scans employed FSE technique, using three echoes. The dose of contrast administered was 0.1 mmol/kg. No adjustment was made in contrast dose for the 3 T scan, nor is this recommended. Intravenous contrast is employed in the postoperative lumbar spine on MR to distinguish scar, which enhances, from recurrent or residual disk material, which does not (when scans are acquired <20 mins postcontrast). Although scar enhances, it does not do so intensely, which has been well appreciated at 1.5 T since approval for this indication in the early 1990s. No published studies exist concerning the relative enhancement of scar at 1.5 versus 3 T. Whatever the improvement at 3 T, if indeed any exists, is well utilized for routine clinical interpretation in the postoperative back.

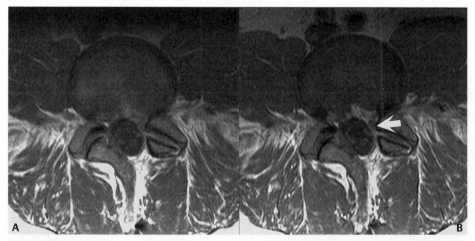

Figure 66–3

67 Spine: Lumbar—Postoperative (Part 2)

Benjamin Hyman and Val M. Runge

Presented in **Fig. 67–1** are postoperative 3 T images of a patient 2 years after L3–L5 laminectomy now with progressively worsening low back pain. A large right paramedian sequestered (free) disk fragment is identified, originating from the L2–3 level, with cephalad migration and thecal sac compression. **Figure 67–1A** is a T2-weighted FSE scan acquired with 4-mm slices, TA 2:44 × 2, and pixel dimensions of 1.1 × 0.5 mm², demonstrating the sequestered fragment (small arrow). The axial T2-weighted FSE scan (TA 1:56 × 2, 0.6 × 0.5 × 4 mm³) shows exquisitely the mild thecal sac compression and intermediate signal intensity of the disk fragment. **(C, D)** present T1-weighted FSE sagittal images acquired with a 4-mm slice thickness and similar spatial resolution. Note the attentive placement of the saturation slabs just anterior to the spine on all sagittal studies, preventing adjacent physiologic motion from entering the field of interest. Marked peripheral enhancement (large arrow) is noted in **Fig. 67–1D** (acquired with fat suppression) after IV gadolinium chelate administration demarcating surrounding granulation tissue. The excellent fat suppression at 3 T allows for exquisite demonstration of the free fragment and resultant thecal sac compression.

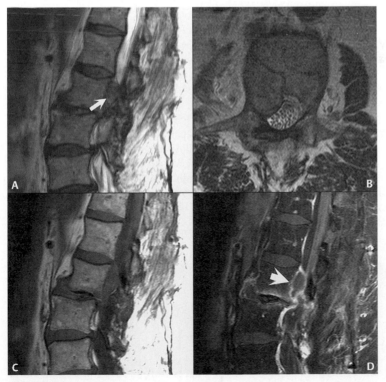

Figure 67–1

68 Spine: Lumbar—Intrathecal (Part 1)

Benjamin Hyman and Val M. Runge

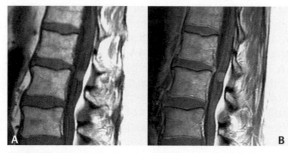

Figure 68–1

The images in this case are from a 75-year-old man with right leg radicular symptoms, exacerbated with walking and prolonged standing. **Figure 68–1** presents postcontrast T1-weighted FSE images from **(A)** 1.5 and **(B)** 3 T demonstrating a small, solitary, well-circumscribed, enhancing intrathecal mass consistent with a schwannoma. Both acquisition time and in-plane resolution for these two studies were similar, and little difference in image quality is seen between the two studies. A very definable difference made with 3 T can be demonstrated when the improved available SNR is put into application with advances in 3D FSE imaging using variable refocusing RF pulses, such as SPACE (see Case 18), along with parallel imaging techniques. This combination has substantially improved the evaluation and diagnosis of small spinal masses. Using SPACE allows for high-resolution 3D images but with lower SAR deposition, which was not the case in previous 2D slice-selective and 3D FSE MR applications. By applying parallel imaging techniques, faster acquisition times can be accomplished comparable with 2D protocols. Unfortunately, the use of parallel imaging is not without some shortcoming, with that being specifically lower SNR. When used in conjunction with 3 T, this loss is mitigated due to the intrinsically higher SNR, leading to excellent high-resolution 3D images with low SAR deposition and acceptable acquisition times. **Figure 68–2** demonstrates T2-weighted FSE sagittal scans acquired at 3 T using SPACE (TR 1500, TE 128, TA 3:29, BW 410, voxel size of $1.2 \times 0.9 \times 1.0$ mm^3).

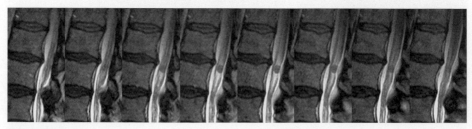

Figure 68–2

69 Spine: Lumbar—Intrathecal (Part 2)

Benjamin Hyman and Val M. Runge

This case presents MR scans from a 39-year-old man with von Hippel-Lindau syndrome who had resection of a pheochromocytoma in the distant past and reports ongoing cervical/upper lumbar back pain, extremity weakness, and paresthesias. In **Fig. 69–1**, axial postcontrast T1-weighted images acquired at 3 T using a 2-mm slice thickness are presented from the cervical **(A)** and lumbar spine **(B to D)**. Depicted are multiple enhancing hemangioblastomas—three involving nerve roots and one involving the conus (arrows). Along with the advent of 3 T, there has been development of multicoil/multielement MR systems that allow for full spine imaging, without manual repositioning or coil reconfiguration between studies, and thus faster overall imaging

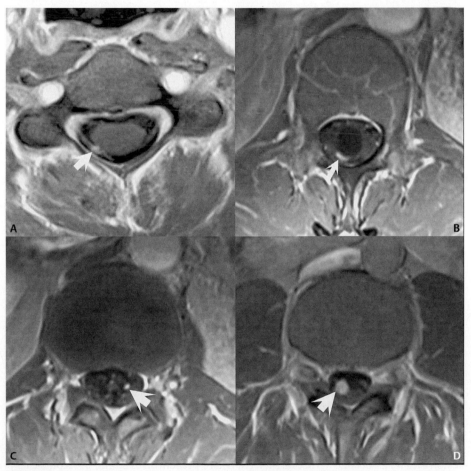

Figure 69–1

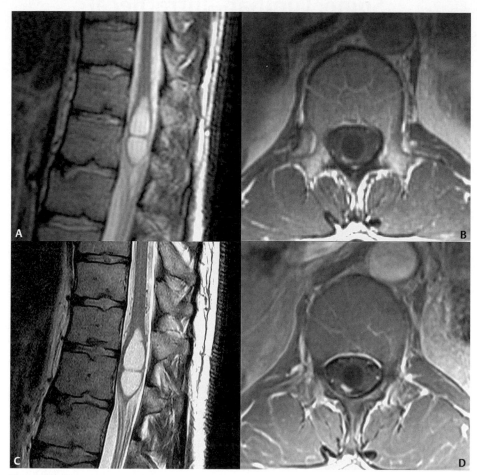

Figure 69–2

times. In this example, the patient's lumbar spine study was performed initially, followed by evaluation of the cervical cord. Between the lumbar and cervical scans, the patient table was repositioned from the operator's console, with less than a second needed to transition between the two studies. **Figure 69–1B** demonstrates a syrinx cavity with enhancement along the right posterior margin, consistent with a hemangioblastoma involving the conus medullaris. **Figures 69–1A, 69–1C,** and **69–1D** depict minute enhancing hemangioblastomas involving (**A**) a dorsal cervical root and (**C, D**) the nerves themselves within the cauda equina. For the first time, 3 T provides the capability of routine 2-mm sections in the spine, whether cervical, thoracic, or lumbar, improving detection of small lesions such as that illustrated. As a correlate, this should dramatically improve the imaging and depiction of leptomeningeal metastatic disease.

Comparison of the lesion in the conus medullaris as depicted at 1.5 and 3 T is illustrated in **Figs. 69–2A** to **69–2D**. Both image sets demonstrate the anatomy of the conus lesion and its associated syrinx further. (**A, B**) are precontrast T2- and postcontrast T1-weighted sections at 1.5 T acquired using 4-mm slices and 0.8 mm² in-plane resolution, (**C, D**) are the equivalent images at 3 T acquired using 2.4-mm slices—in approximately

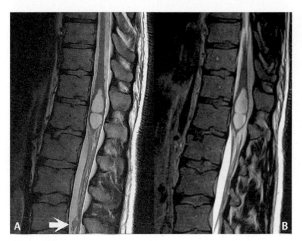

Figure 69–3

the same scan time (~4 min), but with substantially better in-plane spatial resolution (0.3 mm²). With new SAR reduction techniques and thin-section imaging capabilities, 3 T surpasses 1.5 T in the lumbar spine due to improved high-resolution imaging.

Figures 69–3A and **69–3B** compare two different techniques for the acquisition of sagittal thin-section T2-weighted images at 3 T. **(A)** was acquired with FSE technique using 2.4-mm sections (pixel dimensions of 0.6 × 0.5 mm²), demonstrating the conus lesion together with another hemangioblastoma (arrow) further down within the cauda equina. **(B)** depicts the same portion of the lumbar spine acquired using SPACE (a 3D high-resolution low SAR FSE technique). The in-plane resolution for **(B)** is slightly inferior to that in **(A)**, with the SPACE image acquired using a voxel size of 0.9 × 0.9 × 0.9 mm³. However, this permits high-resolution multiplanar reconstructions in any desired orientation. There is a slight difference in tilt between **(A, B)** the two sagittal acquisitions, with the spinal canal slightly oblique relative to the plane of acquisition for the SPACE image. However, this is of little consequence due to the small isometric voxel. **Figure 69–4** shows the reformatting capabilities with SPACE, demonstrating

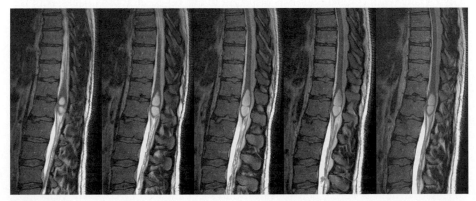

Figure 69–4

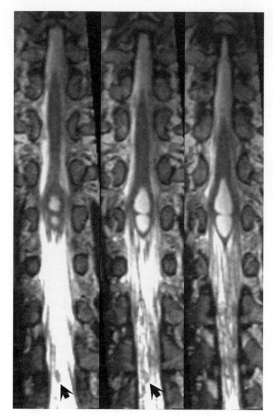

Figure 69–5

contiguous 0.9-mm sagittal sections, now slightly tilted to have the cord in plane. Of note, the small hemangioblastoma located in the lower lumbar canal is visualized on three contiguous slices (as opposed to on one slice of the 2D FSE scan).

The multiplanar reconstruction capabilities using a SPACE acquisition are further demonstrated with coronal reformats displayed in **Fig. 69–5**. On these images, both the lesion within the conus and that lower in the lumbar spine are again visualized.

In summary, the acquisition of high-resolution 3D data sets of the lumbar spine within an acceptable scan time is made possible with 3 T due to the inherent higher SNR. In combination with new multicoil, multielement magnet systems, the entire spine can thus be imaged with high resolution in an acceptable time with no patient manipulation or coil reconfiguration between studies. As SAR reduction strategies come more into practice at 3 T, further gains can be expected in spine imaging, specifically in terms of exam quality and scan time.

Knee: Cartilage
R. Kent Sanders

Diagnosis and staging of various internal derangements is by far the most common purpose of MR imaging of the knee. By virtue of their superior spatial/anatomic resolution, 3 T magnets provide the most accurate and detailed depiction of chondral, subchondral, and ligamentous injuries. At our institution, a standard internal derangement protocol for the knee includes axial proton density with fat saturation (TE 35/TR 3500, 4-mm slice thickness, and 384 × 512 matrix), sagittal proton density without fat saturation (TE 22/TR 3300, 2.5-mm slice thickness, and 384 × 512 matrix), sagittal T2 with fat saturation (TE 65/TR 5500, 2.5-mm slice thickness, and 384 × 512 matrix), coronal T1 without fat saturation (TE 15/TR 550, 3-mm slice thickness, and 288 × 384 matrix), and coronal T2 with fat saturation (TE 65/TR 3500, 3-mm slice thickness, and 256 × 512 matrix).

♦ Cartilage

Patellofemoral dysfunction accounts for a majority of anterior knee pain. Whether from true chondromalacia or adverse biomechanics with patellofemoral instability, patellar cartilage lesions are easily evaluated on axial imaging. FSE proton density sequences, with or without fat saturation, provide excellent resolution of the cartilage surface interface with surrounding joint fluid or adjacent femoral cartilage. **Figure 70–1A** is a non-fat-saturated sagittal image that shows the normal cartilage-fluid signal contrast between the patellar superior pole cartilage and suprapatellar

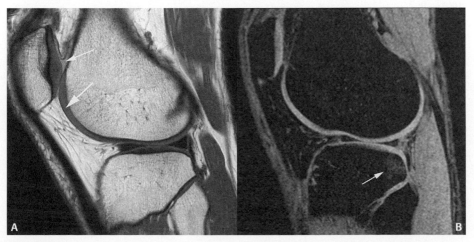

Figure 70–1

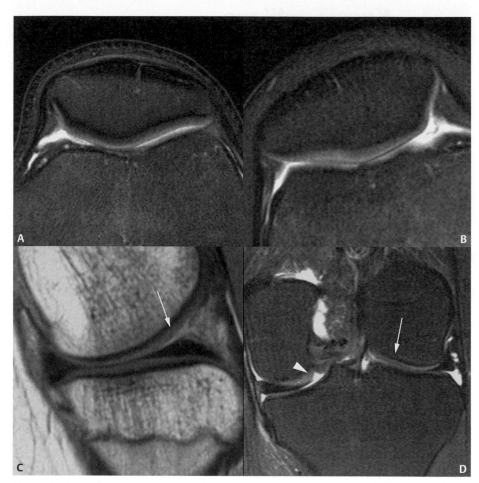

Figure 70–2

recess joint fluid (small arrow). Chemical shift artifact likely contributes to the conspicuity of the cartilage-fat interface of the femoral trochlear cartilage and Hoffa's fat pad (large arrow) as the frequency encoding direction is anterior-posterior. The proton density sequence has the advantage over cartilage dedicated GRE or spoiled GRE techniques **(Fig. 70–1B)** in that it also better depicts fine detail of the intrinsic and extrinsic ligaments and capsule of the knee. The arrow in **Fig. 70–1B** shows the location of a bone bruise associated with a recent anterior cruciate ligament (ACL) tear. The cartilage of the femoral lateral condylar notch and posterior tibial plateau appears normal.

In **Fig. 70–2A,** the superficial tangential zone of collagen in the surface layer of the patellar cartilage can be seen as a discrete low signal line that is often not resolved with 1.5 T imaging. Note the uniform gradation of fluid signal intensity from the transitional layer to the deeper radial layer. The calcified layer is generally not distinguishable from the subchondral bone plate in normal cartilage. Where intact cartilage surfaces abut, the tangential zones are correspondingly twice as apparent due to the apposition of these two dark/low-signal lines. **Figure 70–2B** is an axial proton density image through the patellofemoral joint of a 15-year-old female that illustrates accentuation of the tangential zone contact of the medial patellar facet and femoral trochlea. **Figure 70–2C** shows the same phenomenon within the medial femorotibial compartment, this time on a non-fat-saturated sagittal proton density image. The arrow indicates the location of a subtle disruption of the tangential zone by a superficial chondral lesion with fraying. Note the absence of the fine dark line that normally delineates the cartilage surface. There is also a shallow fissure along the leading edge of the defect. **Figure 70–2D** is a coronal T2 fat-saturated image where the arrow again shows the double tangential zone contact. Compare this to the appearance of the tangential zone along the sharply curving surface of the lateral femoral condyle (arrowhead) where the line is normally not apparent. The fine dark line of the tibial plateau interface with joint fluid of the lateral femorotibial compartment opposite the arrowhead is a good example of a single tangential zone interface with fluid. Accentuation of the black lines of the double tangential zone contact helps to maintain the sensitivity for detecting even superficial cartilage lesions at 3 T. Poor visualization of this line due to magic angle and/or volume averaging effect can occur in predictable locations where the curvature of the articular surface abruptly changes—usually at the margins of the superior and inferior poles of the patella and margins of the femoral condyles as in **Fig. 70–2D**. However, this is generally not a source of confusion in the patellofemoral joint given that most patellar cartilage pathology occurs at or near the apex between the medial and lateral facets and throughout the lateral facet. Sagittal sequences generally show the margins of the superior and inferior poles with better clarity, as they are more perpendicular to the cartilage and subchondral plates of the poles. Patellar lesions limited to these locations can be detected along with the corresponding injuries to the quadriceps and patellar tendons and Hoffa's fat pad attachments by use of the sagittal sequences. **Figures 70–3A** through **70–3D** show a case of chronic patellar tendinosis associated with patellofemoral instability from underlying lateral femoral condylar and trochlear hypoplasia in a 36-year-old male. Note the shallow trochlear groove (normal sulcus angle 146 ± 5 degrees) and dominant lateral patellar facet with rounding of the patellar apex (arrow) in **Fig. 70–3A**. **Figure 70–3B** is an AP radiograph with the knee semiflexed showing the transverse constriction of the hypoplastic lateral condyle (arrows) and the widening of the lateral compartment joint space (arrowhead). **Figure 70–3C** is a sagittal proton density of the same case. The arrowhead shows a focal chondral lesion of the central patellar cartilage with fraying and at least one deep fissure superiorly. The small arrows show small inferior pole patellar enthesophytes while the large arrows point out edema and thickening of the proximal and distal patellar tendon. The fat-saturated axial T2 in **Fig. 70–3D** better shows the thickened fibrotic fibers (arrowheads) of the patellar tendon with centrally located amorphous elevated fluid signal (arrow) possibly reflecting mucoid change from chronic inflammation.

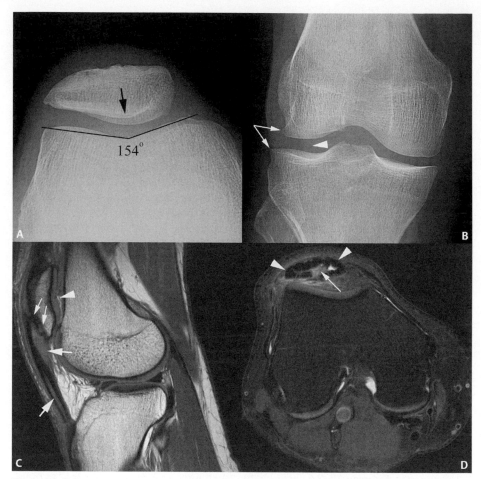

Figure 70–3

Thinning of the articular cartilage can be graded in groups of 1 though 4 with each group representing an additional 25% of thickness lost. **Figure 70–4A** is an axial proton density image with fat saturation where the arrow indicates a focal superficial chondral lesion of the medial patellar facet. Note the loss of the tangential zone dark line and adjacent patch of fibrillated cartilage just anterior to the arrow. **Figure 70–4B** is a sagittal proton density image without fat saturation of the same lesion. The arrow again shows the interface of joint fluid and the fibrillated cartilage.

As normal patellar cartilage is between 3 and 4 mm in thickness, a grade-2 lesion with between 25 and 50% thinning is generally easily distinguished from a grade-3 lesion with between 50 and 75% thinning. **Figure 70–4C** is another axial proton density image with fat saturation that shows an obliquely oriented fissure extending to half of the cartilage thickness. The obliquity of its dissection through the upper layers

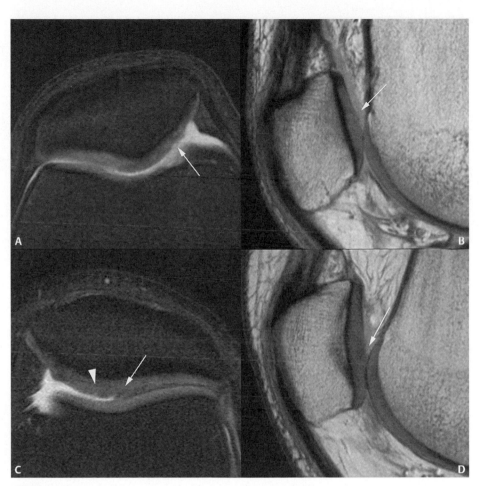

Figure 70–4

of the cartilage suggests that rather than eventually penetrating the calcified layer, this lesion will go on to become a cartilaginous flap. The adjacent arrowhead indicates a small violation of the tangential zone with locally increased intrasubstance fluid signal. **Figure 70–4D** is a sagittal proton density image from the same case showing the open surface of the fissure and inferior oblique dissection (arrow). Engagement of the patella in the sulcus terminale of the femur during extension will open the fissure and propagate the lesion.

Full-thickness lesions that extend to the subchondral plate always result in subchondral edema initially and subchondral fibrocystic degeneration of bone eventually. Full-thickness fissures will have a focal flame-shaped area of edema while larger areas of exfoliation will have edema throughout the width of the exposed subchondral plate. An exception to the latter would be an acute/hyperacute chondral shear injury where cartilage separates along its deep calcified layer leaving

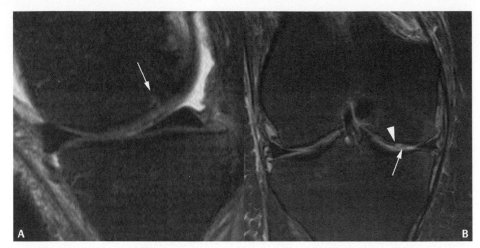

Figure 70–5

the bony subchondral plate intact. **Figure 70–5A** is a sagittal T2-weighted image with fat saturation that shows a minute plume of subarticular edema (arrow) associated with an acute medial femoral condylar impaction injury that focally disrupted the adjacent subchondral plate. **Figure 70–5B** is a coronal T2-weighted image with fat saturation where the arrow indicates the apex of a cartilaginous flap within a more chronic chondral defect of the medial femoral condyle. The arrowhead marks the edge of the chondral defect. Note that the edge of the defect is rounded rather than frayed and shows uniformly low signal, likely representing chondral fibrosis. Marginal spurring attests to chronic osteoarthritis whereas medial compartment marginal edema indicates elevated stress distribution from an incompetent medial meniscus and worsening varus angulation. Contrast the appearance of this chronic chondral lesion to the acutely torn and flipped chondral flap of the medial patellar facet in **Fig. 70–6A**. This is an axial proton density image with fat saturation in an adolescent male who suffered a direct blow to the medial anterior patella. The small arrow indicates a fold in the tangential zone fibers of the cartilage that remain connected to the sheared fragment. The large arrow indicates a focal band of subchondral trabecular impaction. Superficial to this there is a disruption of the subchondral plate. Note the loose fibers of the cartilage transitional zone in between the arrows. There is increased fluid signal in the frayed edges of this defect as apposed to low signal fibrosis found in chronic lesions. The white arrowhead shows the torn fibers of the medial patellofemoral ligament/retinaculum attachment on the medial patella whereas the black arrowhead shows the stump of the torn medial patellar plica. **Figure 70–6B** is an example of full-thickness cartilage exfoliation of the entire lateral patellar facet as shown on routine axial proton density with fat saturation. The subchondral plate

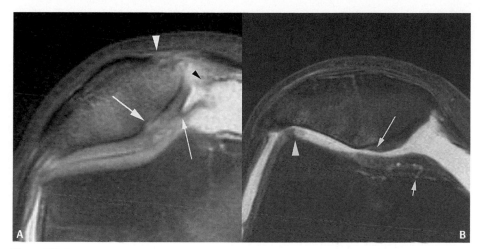

Figure 70–6

is intact. Small plumes of subchondral edema are scattered throughout the length of the defect. The long arrow shows the smooth and slightly fibrotic edge of the apical extent of the patellar defect while the arrowhead shows the sharp nonfibrotic edge of a newer focal full-thickness defect in the superior medial trochlear ridge of the femur. The small arrow shows the transcortical segment of a normal perforator vessel entering the supratrochlear portion of the femoral metaphysis. No cartilage is normally present medially at this level.

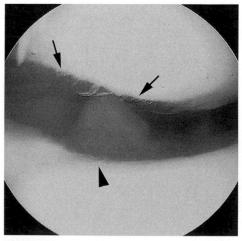

Figure 70–7

Superficial fraying, particularly at the patellar apex is common. **Figure 70–7** is a common arthroscopic appearance of the patellofemoral joint in which there is fine fibrillation of the cartilage surface at the patellar apex and lateral facet (arrows) and a matching area in the sulcus terminale of the femoral trochlea (arrowhead). A focal superficial defect of the cartilage can occasionally lead to intrasubstance edema, or imbibing of joint fluid into the cartilage, resulting in bulging of the overlying surface and an increase in the thickness of the cartilage locally. These lesions are soft to arthroscopic probing and are referred to as chondral blisters. They are equivalent to grade-2 chondromalacia.

Femorotibial cartilage lesions are common in older individuals as a result of osteoarthritis, meniscal degeneration, and incompetence, and in anyone with ACL deficiency, meniscal tear or significant impaction injury. Acute osteochondral impaction fractures, chronic repetitive osteochondral injuries (osteochondrosis dissecans), and subchondral insufficiency fractures are all well demonstrated with the routine internal derangement protocol at 3 T.

71 Knee: Osteochondral Disease

R. Kent Sanders

Acute impaction injury patterns range from isolated chondral destruction, isolated subchondral bone bruises and/or fractures, to any combination of these injuries. The degree of bony penetration and trabecular disruption correlates directly with the amount of energy transfer and the area over which the impulse is inflicted across the joint surface. Edema associated with energy dispersal in bone generally assumes a hemispherical geometry with the point of impact being demarcated by the most intense edema. By the time imaging is obtained, there is generally a second pattern of vasogenic edema that surrounds the dilated capsular perforator vessels that supply the injured bone. This pattern is perivascular in distribution and therefore follows a vascular territory that in the femur and tibia is wedge-like in morphology. With subchondral trabecular fracturing, there is a discrete low-signal zone marking the compression of the trabecula and exclusion of marrow fat. **Figures 71–1A** to **71–1D** show a typical acute osteochondral impaction fracture involving the anterolateral tibial plateau. **Figure 71–1A** is an axial proton density image with fat saturation in which the arrowheads outline the hemisphere of impaction edema or bruising deep to the zone of trabecular impaction. The arrow shows the perivascular accumulation of vasogenic edema caused by dilatation of an adjacent intraosseous arteriole. **Figure 71–1B** is a coronal T1 image illustrating the usefulness of T1 imaging in displaying the zone of subchondral trabecular impaction. Arrowheads mark the edges of the fracture. The thin cartilage of the anterior tibia is not as well seen as with proton density imaging. **Figure 71–1C** is a sagittal proton density image where the cartilage/subchondral plate interface is much better appreciated. A subtle depression of the subchondral plate is visible (arrowhead) despite no apparent fissuring of the overlying cartilage. In **Figure 71–1C**, there are concentric low-signal linear arcs (arrows) within the trabecular bone far below the zone of obvious trabecular compression that mark the limits of the subchondral fragment illustrated in **Fig. 71–1B**. This may reflect lesser degrees of trabecular injury/fracture and attests to the great amount of energy transmitted into the tibia as the result of its being directly hit by a fellow football player's helmet during a tackle. **Figure 71–1D** is a coronal T2 image with fat saturation that was obtained just posterior to the impaction fracture. The arrow indicates a dilated tibial perforator vessel while the arrowheads show nondilated normal-appearing tibial and femoral perforators. Note the irregular morphology of the deeper perivascular edema on the T2 image. There is, however, lack of trabecular detail on the heavily T2-weighted image.

With uncomplicated healing, this low-signal zone remodels into a normal trabecular pattern. In cases where the subchondral bone goes on to infarction, this subchondral fragment my resorb and get replaced with scar tissue or form subchondral cysts/geodes. In some instances, the fragment may stabilize and act as in an in situ graft that results in focal hypertrophy of the subchondral bone. These chronic injuries can be recognized by their rounded, incongruent margins that tend to protrude beyond the normal contour of the subchondral plate. They are frequently associated with fibrosis or absence of the overlying cartilage and may also have internal or marginal cystic degeneration. As a result of degeneration/arthritis, chronic lesions may

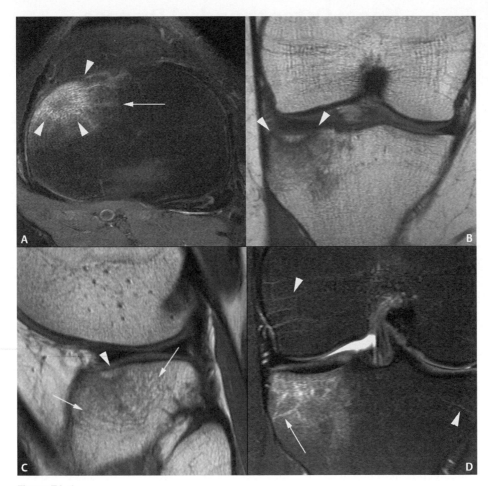

Figure 71–1

remain hyperemic and edematous. **Figure 71–2A** is a sagittal proton density image of a healing osteochondrosis dissecans (OCD) lesion in the medial femoral condyle of a skeletally immature male with multiple lesions. Note the rounded and protuberant contour of the subchondral plate along the leading edge (white arrow) and fibrosis in the posterior edge (arrowhead). The black arrow indicates a smaller adjacent tibial lesion. **Figure 71–2B** is a coronal T2 image with fat saturation through the same lesion. The small arrow indicates the zone of demarcation between the donor site and the remodeling trabecular impaction zone. Increased fluid signal in the fragment and within the adjacent bone (large arrow) reflects invading granulation tissue and potential reincorporation of the fragment. Note vasodilatation and edema along the capsular perforator vessels of the femoral condyle (arrowheads). **Figure 71–2C** is a coronal T2 with fat saturation through the lateral femoral condyle of the same knee. The arrow shows sclerosis in this OCD lesion with a less T2-intense halo (arrowhead) deep to this nearly healed smaller and shallower defect. **Figure 71–2D** is a sagittal proton density

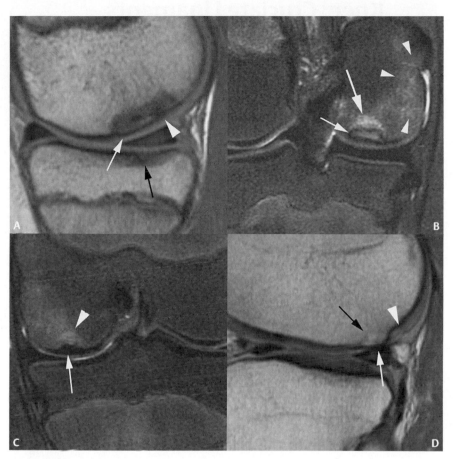

Figure 71–2

image in a different patient that shows a completely healed lesion that is particularly hypertrophic and protuberant. The black arrow shows the remnants of the trabecular impaction zone. The white arrow indicates the absence of cartilage that normally separates the surface of the condyle from the adjacent meniscus. Note the change in signal intensity within fibrocartilage/scar tissue deposited between the posterior edge of the lesion and the remaining posterior condylar cartilage (arrowhead). The termination of the posterior condylar cartilage tangential zone is visible at this interface.

72 Knee: Cruciate Ligaments
R. Kent Sanders

Sagittal oblique 2.5-mm sequences along the plane of the anterior cruciate ligament (ACL) typically yield three to four images of the ACL, with the first medial image depicting the anterior band in isolation from the intermediate fibers. Normal ACL morphology includes distinct fiber condensations along the anterior and posterior bands with varying degrees of synovial tissue and fat separating the striations of the intermediate fibers. The anterior band should be straight from origin to insertion and generally will not contact the roof of the intercondylar notch. There are degrees of apparent mild laxity particularly in adolescents with gracile body morphotypes. **Figures 72–1A** and **72–1B** are sagittal proton density images depicting normal variation in ACL fiber densities. In **Fig. 72–1A**, distinct anterior and posterior band fiber condensations (large and small arrows, respectively) are visible against a paucity of intermediate fibers in this 15-year-old girl. **Figure 72–1B** shows a more robust anterior band (large arrow) with very dense intermediate fibers (small arrow), and a poorly defined posterior band tibial attachment (white arrowhead) in this 40-year-old man. Note the straightness of the anterior bands and the small gap separating the anterior bands from the intercondylar notches (black arrowheads).

Laxity of the anterior band (if it angles around the roof of the intercondylar notch) and replacement of the intermediate fiber stripes with poorly defined low signal indicates an old partial tear and fibrosis of the ACL, while acute tears have intrasubstance edema or hemorrhage. **Figure 72–2A** is a sagittal proton density image of a chronically ACL deficient knee. Arrows indicate the laxity of the ACL with impingement along the roof of the intercondylar notch of the femur. Note the loss of the normal striated appearance of the intermediate fibers (arrowhead) and the thickness of the anterior band. **Figure 72–2B** is a fat-saturated T2 through the same location that shows the

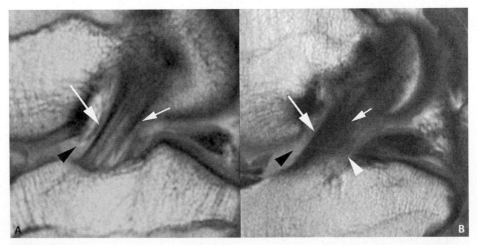

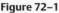
Figure 72–1

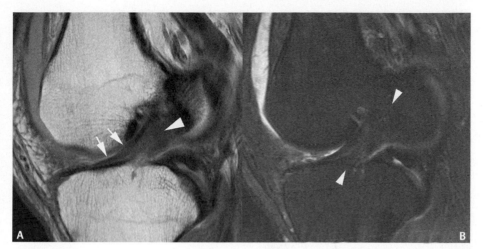

Figure 72–2

lack of edema in both the ACL and the adjacent bony attachments (arrowheads). Compare this appearance to **Fig. 72–3A** (a sagittal T2 image with fat saturation) that shows an acute intrasubstance partial tear of the ACL. There is increased T2 signal among the intermediate fibers with bowing of the fibers and expansion of the cruciate synovial jacket due to intracruciate hemorrhage. The arrow in **Fig. 72–3A** shows bowing of the anterior band around the intercondylar notch and loss of the normal gap beneath the intercondylar notch. Intraosseous vasodilatation (arrowhead) is an additional sign of acuity. The ACL fibers can still be traced from femur to tibia. The effusion is relatively small because the cruciate bleeding is mostly contained in the extrasynovial space (arrowheads in **Fig. 72–3B**, axial proton density with fat saturation). Accentuated hooking of an otherwise normal-appearing posterior cruciate ligament (PCL) may accompany this finding **(Fig. 72–3C)**. Anterior drawer laxity with a firm endpoint is evident clinically.

Isolated rupture of the anterior band generally occurs at the femoral or tibial attachments. Acute injuries will display associated localized bone marrow edema at the corresponding bony attachment sites. These same areas of edema frequently mature into intraosseous fibrocystic changes in the setting of chronic injuries. **Figure 72–4** is a coronal T2 image with fat saturation that shows subarticular/intraosseous cystic degeneration (arrowheads) of the tibial intercondylar eminence associated with a chronic partial tear of the ACL. An arrow marks the wavy detached ACL fiber. Chronic partial ACL injuries can also result in the development of intracruciate synovial cysts that can present as low-grade deep knee pain with restricted motion.

Complete ACL tears occur at the femoral attachment or midsubstance of the ligament. Disorganized and frayed tissue with marked edema and hemorrhage are easily detected in the acute setting along with marked hooking of the PCL from anterior translation of the tibia. **Figures 72–5A** and **72–5B** are sagittal proton density images of similar proximal complete tears of the ACL. **Figure 72–5A** is an acute tear in which the retracted ACL fibers are swollen and hemorrhagic (white arrow), and there is a large joint effusion/hemarthrosis that anteriorly displaces the apex of Hoffa's fat (black arrow). In **Fig. 72–5B**, the chronically torn and retracted ACL stump has a discrete

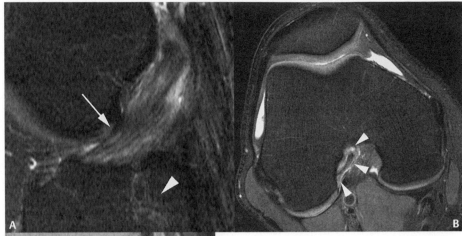

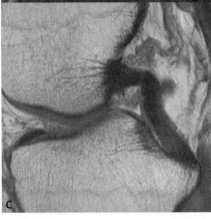

Figure 72–3

low-signal fibrotic appearance without edema (white arrow) and is surrounded by adherent fat rather than fluid (black arrow).

In the case of flail injuries of the knee (ejected motor vehicle accidents and downhill skiing), PCL tears may simultaneously occur as the result of transient anterior and posterior subluxation/dislocation. Bone bruise patterns often elucidate the mechanism of injury. Lateral femoral condylar bruises/osteochondral impaction fractures and posterior tibial plateau bruises/impaction fractures typify ACL injuries along with lateral greater than medial posterior meniscal tears, medial collateral ligament tears, and medial retinaculum strains. Lateral tibial rim (Segond) fractures and lateral collateral/conjoined ligament tears are uncommon in our experience.

The anterolateral and posteromedial fascicles of the PCL and variations of the posterior meniscofemoral ligaments are best demonstrated on axial images. **Figures 72–6A** through **72–6F** show normal thin and robust PCLs, respectively. **Figures 72–6A** and **72–6B** are axial proton density images through the femoral origins of the PCL in a 27-year-old woman and 40-year-old man, respectively. Both images are oriented to represent a right knee. Note the discrete yet wavy fiber definition in **Fig. 72–6A** (arrow) versus the denser

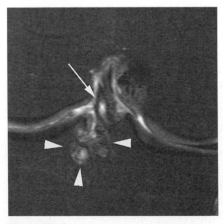

Figure 72–4

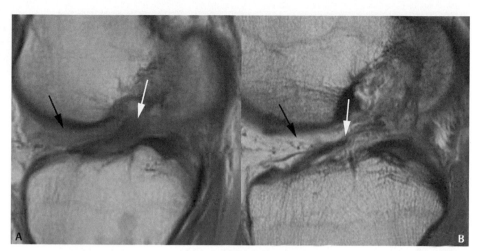

Figure 72–5

and less discrete fiber definition in **Fig. 72–6B** (arrow). Arrowheads mark the proximal ACLs in both cases. **Figures 72–6C** and **72–6D** are from the same series closer to the femorotibial joint line. Arrows indicate slight indentations of the PCL cross-sectional contour that mark the abutment of the anterolateral (to the viewer's left) and posteromedial fascicles (to the viewer's right). As with the proximal images, differences in fiber conspicuity persist to the tibial attachment. **Figures 72–6E** and **72–6F** are sagittal proton density images from the same individuals. Note the straighter contour and thinner caliber in **Fig. 72–6E**. The black arrow indicates a relatively large meniscofemoral ligament of Humphrey passing anterior to the PCL. The white arrow indicates the posterior capsule of the knee that is thin and uniform with little or no indication of the oblique popliteal ligament fibers. In **Fig. 72–6F**, the PCL is less straight and uniformly thicker. The arrow indicates a fold in the cruciate synovial jacket that is excluding joint fluid (brighter signal below) from the pericruciate extrasynovial space. The arrowhead indicates focal thickening of the posterior joint capsule due to the fiber contributions of the oblique popliteal ligament.

Stretch injuries/partial tears of the PCL are seen with low-velocity hyperextension injuries (especially in older individuals) and should be suspected if there is abnormal hooking of the PCL despite a normal-appearing ACL. Kissing contusions of the anterior femoral condyles and tibial plateau may be present in an acute injury along with strain or rupture of the posterior capsule/oblique popliteal ligament. Hyperextension-related isolated tears of the posteromedial fascicle may cause increased fluid signal and fusiform enlargement of the PCL without significant hooking or apparent laxity as the intact posterior medial fascicle is much larger and less affected by extension. **Figure 72–7A** is an axial proton density image with fat saturation that shows a posteromedial fascicle tear in the right knee of a young adult athlete. The arrows indicate the division between the anterolateral fascicle, which is dark and normal in cross section, and the torn posteromedial fascicle, which is enlarged and heterogeneously increased in fluid signal. **Figure 72–7B** is a coronal T2 image with fat saturation of the same case. The arrow indicates the normal-appearing

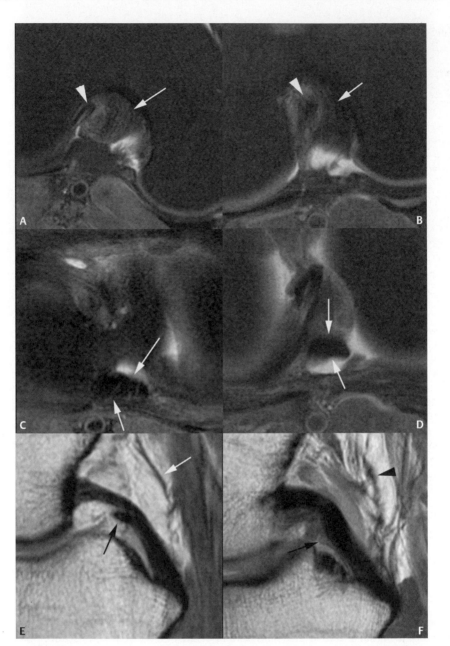

Figure 72–6

anterolateral fascicle. The large arrowhead points to fiber separation at the interface of the fascicles. The torn posteromedial fascicle forms the bulk of the amorphous tissue below. The small arrowhead indicates the normal fibers of the anterior band of the ACL that is being medially displaced by the swollen PCL.

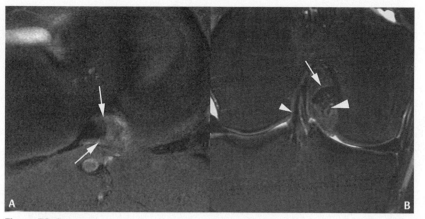

Figure 72–7

Complete disruption of the PCL occurs with posterior knee dislocation and is frequently associated with a medial gastrocnemius tendon tear. This should prompt an inspection of the popliteal artery for pseudoaneurysm or dissection. Arterial spasm is frequently found. **Figure 72–8A** is another axial proton density fat-saturated image of a right knee, this time demonstrating complete disruption of the PCL. The arrows indicate the outline of the massively expanded fascicles. There is hemorrhage throughout the PCL with complete loss of the fiber architecture internally. In **Fig. 72–8B,** the same tear is illustrated in the sagittal plane with a fat-saturated T2 sequence. Arrowheads indicate the separated fascicle tracts proximally. The arrow shows disrupted fibers at the level of the tear, from which the image in **Fig. 72–8A** was obtained.

Dedicated 1-mm sagittal proton density images of the reconstructed cruciate ligament can be added to the routine knee protocol for the evaluation of graft failure. Anterior impingement and percentage of graft fiber disruption are readily depicted, as is the relationship of the graft fibers to interference screws in cases of early failure

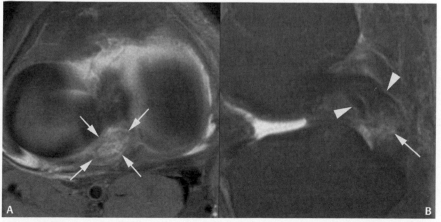

Figure 72–8

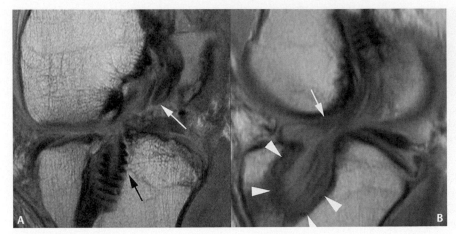

Figure 72–9

from graft laceration. **Figure 72–9A** is a sagittal proton density image showing complete disruption of an ACL graft. The white arrow indicates the retracted graft stump that has detached from the tibial tunnel. There is little susceptibility artifact due to the use of a bioabsorbable interference screw (black arrow). **Figure 72–9B** is a 1.5 T sagittal proton density image of a case of cystic degeneration of an ACL graft. Detached fibers have herniated into the anterior intercondylar region and there is anterior translation of the tibial resulting in graft impingement along the roof of the intercondylar notch (arrow). There is also marked resorption of bone along the tibial tunnel (arrowheads). Note the absence of trabecular and articular surface detail when compared with the 3 T image in **Fig. 72–9A**.

Knee: Menisci/Meniscal Ligaments
R. Kent Sanders

3 T imaging produces higher-resolution images of intrameniscal anatomy (as compared with 1.5 T), particularly of the meniscocapsular junction and meniscofemoral ligaments. **Figures 73–1A** and **73–1B** are coronal T2 images with fat saturation of the right knee of a 15-year-old boy and 34-year-old man, respectively. Arrowheads mark the medial capsule attachments that define the medial gutters. **Figures 73–1C** and **73–1D** are sagittal proton density images through the lateral menisci of the same individuals. Note the simple meniscocapsular strut configuration of the younger individual in **Fig. 73–1C** (arrows) compared with that in the older individual shown in **Fig. 73–1D**. Arrowheads indicate the popliteus tendon within the lateral meniscal popliteus hiatus.

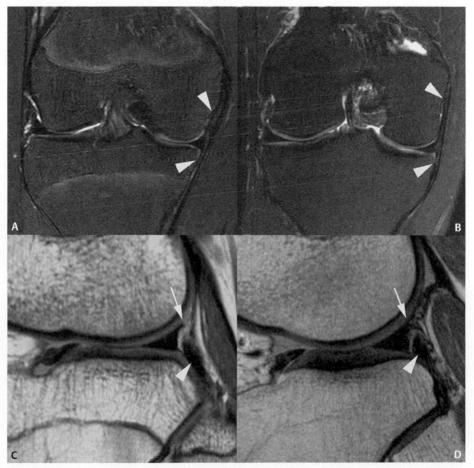

Figure 73–1

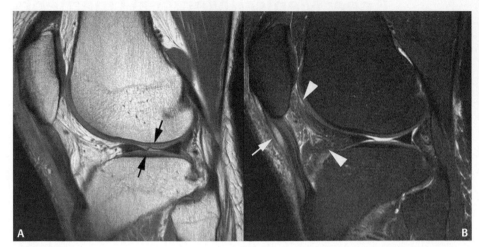

Figure 73–2

Meniscal flounce is a term that describes a wavy contour to the free edge of a meniscus. It has been described as a normal variant and also as a subtle sign of meniscal pathology causing laxity of the circumferential fiber tracts. **Figures 73–2A** and **73–2B** are sagittal proton density and fat-saturated T2 images of a knee with an acute partial tear of the patellar tendon. In **Fig. 73–2A**, the wavy flounce of the lateral meniscus is well shown (arrows). No intrinsic pathology of the lateral meniscus was found in this case. **Figure 73–2B** shows the extensive edema within the patellar tendon (arrow) and within Hoffa's fat pad (arrowheads). It is possible that in this case, the edema may have induced slight posterior displacement of the anterior horn of the lateral meniscus resulting in compression of its normal ringlike structure and thus causing the flounce of the free edge.

Acute compression injuries of the menisci result in "contusion" patterns of fluid signal within the substance of the meniscus. This is characterized by intermediate fluid signal that generally includes the vascular zone and therefore may reflect intrasubstance hemorrhage. Its geometry is nonlinear or amorphous and may or may not extend to the articular surface. Unlike mucoid degeneration, it should be low in T1 signal intensity. **Figures 73–3A** and **73–3B** are sagittal proton density and coronal T2 with fat saturation images, respectively, from a young athlete who sustained an impaction injury to the knee. In addition to a medial femoral condylar cartilage injury (large arrowhead), there is a medial meniscal contusion/crush injury with deformity of the posterior horn (arrow in **Fig. 73–3A**) and extensive nonlinear intrasubstance fluid signal (large arrows in **Fig. 73–3B**). Note in **Fig. 73–3B** the excellent depiction of the meniscofemoral ligament of Wrisberg (small arrowhead) and the lateral meniscocapsular struts outlining the popliteus hiatus highlighted here with the small arrows. Vertical tears of the menisci follow the radial or longitudinal fiber tracts and therefore are generally seen in younger individuals without mucoid degeneration. **Figure 73–4A** is a sagittal proton density image that shows a typical vertically oriented radial tear of the lateral meniscus (arrow). **Figure 73–4B** is a fortuitous axial proton density image with fat saturation that shows the radial orientation of the tear (arrowheads) in the

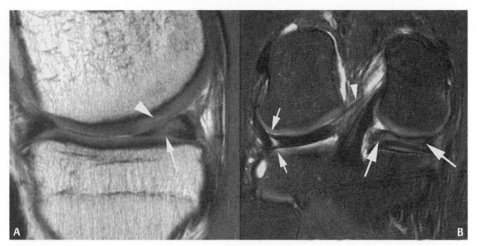

Figure 73–3

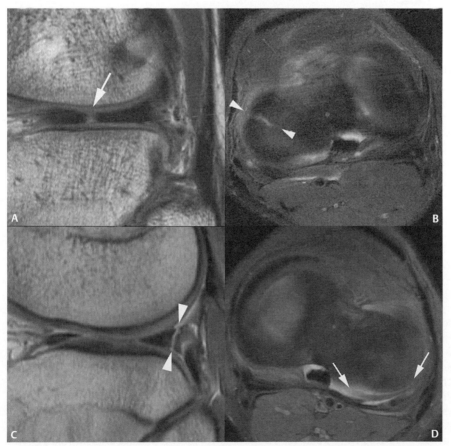

Figure 73–4

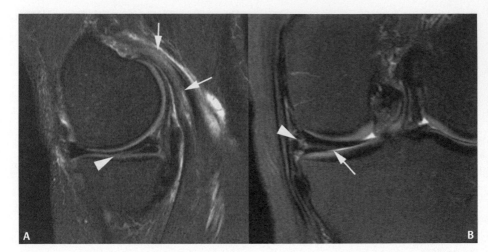

Figure 73–5

same case. **Figures 73–4C** and **73–4D** are similar sequences of a vertical tear in the lateral meniscus that is longitudinally oriented. Arrowheads in **Fig. 73–4C** show the peripheral location tear through the posterior horn of the lateral meniscus while the arrows in **Fig. 73–4D** show the same tear's longitudinal extent. Horizontal tears are separations of the superior and inferior fiber tracts of the meniscus that usually involve delamination of the meniscus at or near the central fibrovascular core. Anterior cruciate deficient knees, particularly in older individuals with early mucoid degeneration, commonly display this tear pattern. **Figure 73–5A** is a fat-saturated sagittal T2 image showing a medial meniscal horizontal oblique tear (arrowhead) that extends to the inferior articular surface of the posterior horn. A more recent injury caused the partial tear of the medial gastrocnemius tendon (arrows). **Figure 73–5B** is a fat-saturated coronal T2 image of another horizontal oblique tear (arrow) this time extending from the inferior articular surface of the body of the medial meniscus to the meniscocapsular junction along the central fibrovascular core of the meniscus (arrowhead).

When the tear dissects anteriorly and posteriorly, the superior portion will become mechanically unstable and will displace or flip medially as a flap if one end remains attached or as a bucket handle if both ends remain attached. **Figures 73–6A** and **73–6B** are sagittal proton density and coronal T2 with fat saturation images of a flipped bucket handle tear of the medial meniscus. The arrows indicate the flipped meniscal fragment in both images while the arrowhead in **Fig. 73–6B** shows the remaining peripheral midbody extent of the causative horizontal meniscal tear. The small arrow in **Fig. 73–6A** shows the twisted connection between the donor portion of the anterior horn and the flipped fragment.

Prior assertions that the presence of a parameniscal cyst implies the presence of a meniscal tear are borne out by the frequent visualization of subtle communications between cysts and adjacent meniscal tears that may have gone previously undetected at 1.5 T. **Figures 73–7A** and **73–7B** are sagittal proton density and coronal T2 with fat saturation images of the same chronically ACL deficient knee shown in **Fig. 72–5B**.

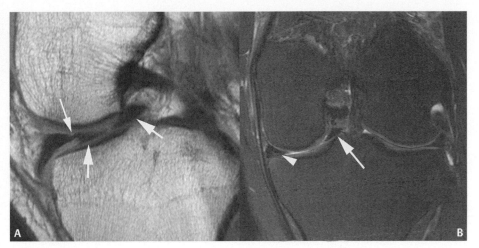

Figure 73–6

The arrow indicates the presence of a small dissecting parameniscal cyst within the meniscocapsular junction of the posterior horn of the lateral meniscus. The multidirectional linear defects adjacent to the cyst (arrowheads in **Fig. 73–7A**) are much less apparent on the coronal T2 sequence. Nonvisualization of a communicating tear raises the possibility of a residual parameniscal cyst adjacent to a healed tear. These cyst-associated tears are frequently intimately apposed with a horizontal orientation that exits the periphery of the disk along the central fibrovascular core of the red zone. The tendency of horizontal tears to appose during weight bearing, along with their long plane of dissection, may enhance their ability to function as a one-way pump of joint fluid into the meniscocapsular junction and thus form parameniscal cysts.

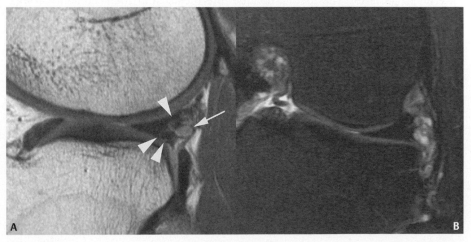

Figure 73–7

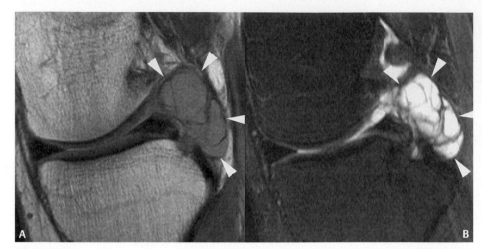

Figure 73–8

Figures 73–8A and **73–8B** are sagittal proton density and fat-saturated T2 images showing a large medial posterior root parameniscal cyst (arrowheads). Note the multiple fine internal septations that typify synovial cysts.

Enhanced visualization of collagen fiber tracts has also resulted in the more frequent detection of meniscal ligament variants such as the anterior lateral meniscocruciate ligament shown in **Fig. 73–9**. White arrows show the anterior horn peripheral fiber tracts separating from the meniscus and blending into the anterior band fibers of the ACL rather than traversing the knee to form the transverse meniscal ligament, which was absent in this case. The top six images **(Figs. 73–9A** to **73–9F)** are sagittal proton density images moving lateral to medial, while the bottom three images **(Figs. 73–9G** to **73–9I)** are coronal fat-saturated T2 going anterior to posterior. The medial oblique intermeniscal or meniscomeniscal ligament and its relationship to the meniscofemoral ligament of Humphrey are shown in **Fig. 73–10**. **Figures 73–10A** and **73–10B** are sequential axial proton density images with fat saturation that first show the meniscofemoral ligament of Humphrey fibers (arrow) passing anteriorly to the anterolateral fascicles of the PCL. In **Fig. 73–10B**, the small arrowhead indicates the remaining meniscofemoral ligament fibers prior to their convergence with the medial oblique intermeniscal fiber tract. The remaining images of **Fig. 73–10C** through **73–10I** are sequential fat-saturated coronal T2 images that progress from anterior to posterior. The arrows indicate the path of the medial oblique intermeniscal ligament as it traverses the anterior cruciate ligament and intracruciate extrasynovial space before attaching to the posterior horn of the lateral meniscus. The persistent median infrapatellar plica can mimic the anterior meniscocruciate ligament as it attaches in the roof of the

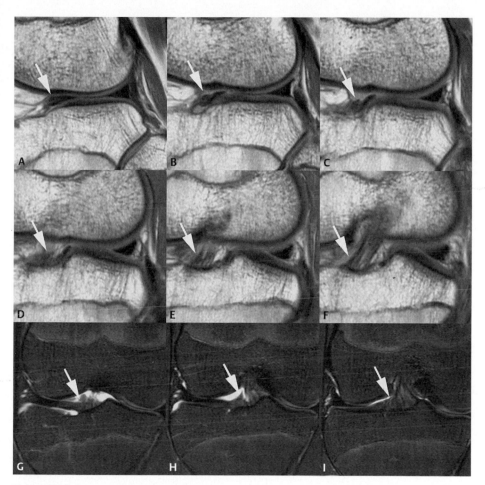

Figure 73–9

intercondylar notch and can intimately parallel the anterior band of the ACL, giving the appearance of attaching to it. **Figures 73–11A** and **73–11B** are sequential sagittal proton density images of a persistent median infrapatellar plica. Arrows mark the extension of the central fibrovascular core of the apex of Hoffa's fat pad into the roof of the intercondylar notch. In this case, there is clear separation of the plica from the synovial jacket of the ACL. The fat pad is draped over the transverse ligament (arrowhead). The transverse ligament does not contribute to the anterior band of the ACL.

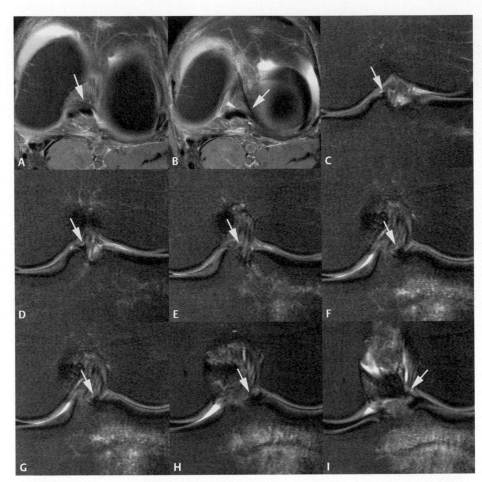

Figure 73–10

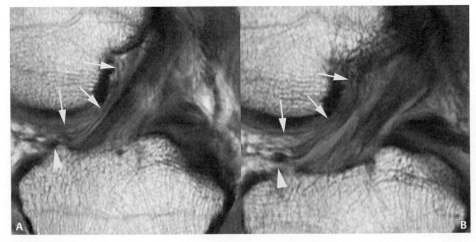

Figure 73–11

74 Knee: Collateral Ligament Complexes

R. Kent Sanders

Axial and coronal sequences best depict the medial and collateral ligaments and their neighboring structures that constitute the collateral complexes. The medial collateral complex includes the crural fascia, the longitudinal and oblique medial collateral ligaments (MCL), the medial capsule, and to a lesser extent the meniscal and capsular attachments of the semimembranosus tendon. The investing fibers of the extensor retinaculum, particularly the medial patellofemoral ligament, are well shown with axial proton density sequences. **Figures 74–1A** and **74–1B** are fat-saturated axial proton density images through the superior and middle third of the medial complex, respectively. **Figure 74–1A** shows the relationship of the medial patellofemoral ligament component of the patellar retinaculum (large arrow) to the longitudinal (superficial) medial collateral ligament (large arrowhead) as well as the crural fascia continuation of the retinaculum (small arrow) and the underlying oblique (deep) medial collateral ligament (small arrowhead). **Figure 74–1B** shows the more distinct divisions of the MCL (the large arrowhead indicates the longitudinal component and the small arrowhead indicates the oblique component) and the extremely thin middle retinaculum (arrow). **Figures 74–2A** through **74–2C** are coronal T1 images through the medial collateral complex progressing from anterior to posterior. In **Fig. 74–2A**, the medial patellofemoral ligament (arrow) passes superficial to the anterior margin of the longitudinal component of the MCL (arrowhead). The adductor magnus tendon (small arrow) attaches to the medial femoral epicondyle proximal to the MCL origin. In **Fig. 74–2B**, the crural fascia continuation of the medial patellofemoral ligament (large arrow) and middle patellar retinaculum (small arrow) are indicated superficial to the thick anterior margin of the longitudinal MCL (arrowhead). The large arrow in **Fig. 74–2C** shows the crural fascia separated from the MCL by fat. The large arrowhead

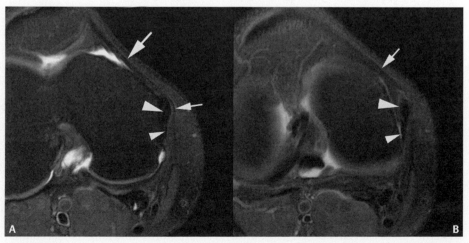

Figure 74–1

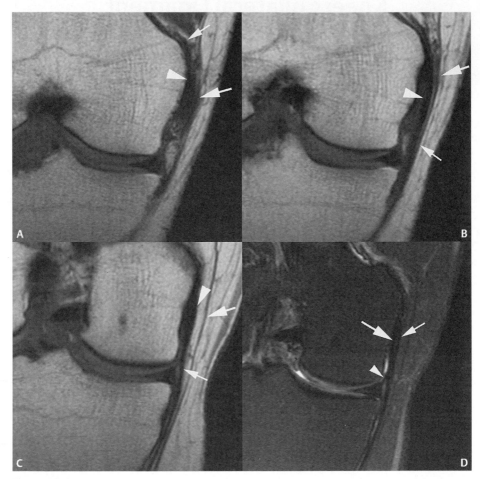

Figure 74–2

shows the posterior extent of the longitudinal component of the MCL. The small arrow shows the deeper anterior margin of the oblique component. **Figure 74–2D** is a fat-saturated coronal T2 that shows a fine T2 signal stripe that marks the boundary between the longitudinal (small arrow) and oblique (large arrow) components of the MCL. The arrowhead indicates the meniscofemoral ligament component of the medial capsule. Its attachment to the femur forms the superior medial gutter and forms the deepest ligamentous layer of the medial collateral complex.

Because of their intimate proximity and possible interconnection to the MCL, medial patellofemoral ligament and retinaculum tears are frequently associated with injury to the underlying anterior and proximal fibers of the MCL. **Figure 74–3A** is a 1.5 T fat-saturated axial proton density image showing an extensive medial collateral complex injury that includes rupture of the medal patellofemoral ligament with delamination from the rest of the retinaculum (large arrowhead), rupture of the longitudinal component of the MCL with intraligamentous hemorrhage (small arrow), and rupture and

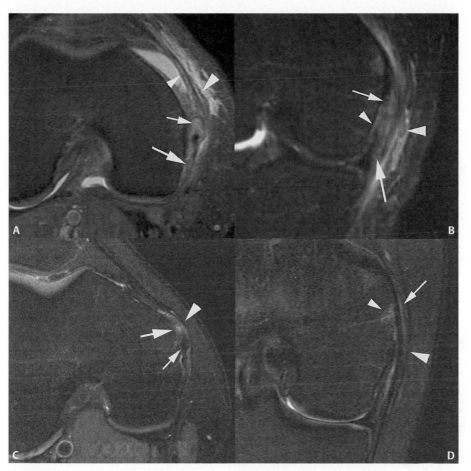

Figure 74–3

retraction of the oblique component of the MCL (large arrow). The small arrowhead indicates the medial patellar plica that appears more conspicuous as it is separated from the retinacular fibers by intracapsular edema. **Figure 74–3B** is a 1.5 T fat-saturated coronal T2 image of the same case that shows discontinuity of the meniscofemoral capsular ligament (small arrowhead), longitudinal (small arrow) and oblique (large arrow) MCL fibers, and laxity/delamination of the crural fascia continuation of the retinaculum (large arrowhead). **Figures 74–3C** and **74–3D** are 3 T images from a nonsurgical focal grade-2 tear of the proximal anterior fibers of the longitudinal component of the MCL. In **Fig. 74–3C**, the large arrow indicates edema and enlargement of the anterior 50% of the longitudinal fibers. The small arrow shows the normal-appearing posterior half. The arrowhead indicates the displaced but intact retinaculum. **Figure 74–3D** is a fat-saturated coronal T2 from the same case obtained just posterior to the swollen portion of the anterior longitudinal fibers. The small arrowhead indicates adjacent bone edema. The arrow shows a small amount of edema tracking posteriorly between the longitudinal fibers and the intact crural fascia (large arrowhead).

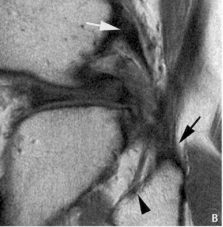

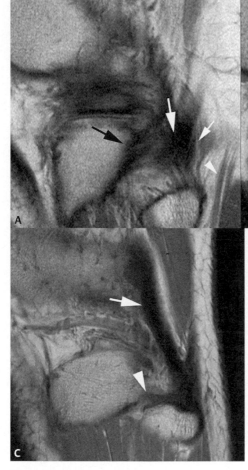

Figure 74–4

The lateral collateral ligament (LCL) and the biceps femoris are the most superficial and largest components of the posterolateral corner ligamentous complex of the knee. The convergence of the biceps and LCL as they attach to the lateral proximal tibia forms the conjoined tendon. The conjoined tendon is far from simple, being formed from the anterior and direct arms of the long head of the biceps, the direct arm of the short head of the biceps, and fibular attachment of the LCL. The anterior arm of the short biceps attaches to the anterolateral tibial metaphysis just below the joint line. This constitutes the anterior oblique fibers of the conjoined tendon and is responsible for the Segond fracture that accompanies ACL tears. **Figures 74–4A** through **74–4C** are sagittal oblique proton density images of the superficial lateral knee. **Figure 74–4A** shows the anterior oblique fibers of the anterior arm of the short head of the biceps femoris attaching to the tibia (black arrow). The anterior arm (white large arrow) and direct arm (small white arrow) of the long head of the biceps femoris have a more vertical path and attach more superficially on the lateral fibular head. The small arrowhead indicates the deep and superficial branches of the common peroneal nerve. These are usually well demonstrated at 3 T on both axial and sagittal proton density sequences. **Figure 74–4B** is 2 mm medial to the image in **Fig. 74–4A** and shows the deeper layers of the biceps tendons. The black arrowhead shows a few remaining fascicles of the anterior arm of the long head of the biceps. The black arrow indicates the direct arm of the short head of the biceps while the white arrow shows the proximal portion of the LCL reaching toward the deep surface of the short head. **Figure 74–4C** is a fortuitous image through the entire length of a

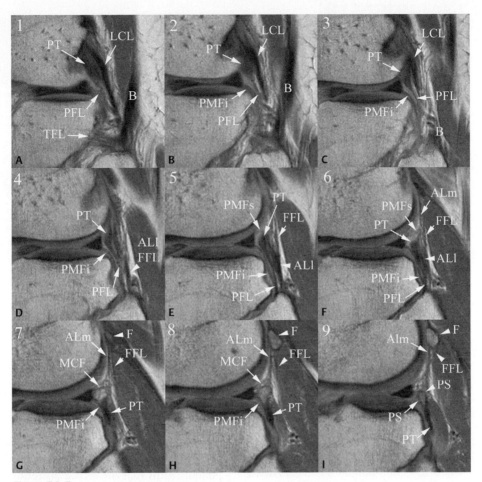

Figure 74–5

robust, and possibly fibrotic, LCL (arrow) in a different knee. Note the lack of striations and layering in the conjoined tendon part of the lateral collateral ligament in this individual. The arrowhead shows the transversely oriented fibers of the anterior proximal tibiofibular ligament.

The tip of the fibular styloid gives rise to the thin capsular ligaments of the posterolateral corner. From superficial to deep these are the fabellofibular ligament, arcuate ligament, popliteofibular ligament, and popliteomeniscal fascicles that form the lateral anchor of the popliteus hiatus of the lateral meniscus. The latter fascicles are contiguous with the meniscocapsular fascicles or struts that form the medial extent of the popliteus hiatus. **Figure 74–5** is a panel of sequential sagittal oblique proton density images through the posterolateral corner of a knee with a fabella. The images progress from lateral to medial and begin at the deep margin of the LCL and biceps tendon (B). The proximal tibiofibular ligament (TFL) marks the sagittal oblique plane between the large superficial collateral ligaments and the deeper capsular ligaments. The path of the popliteus tendon (PT) is paralleled by the popliteofibular ligament (PFL) that shares a common attachment

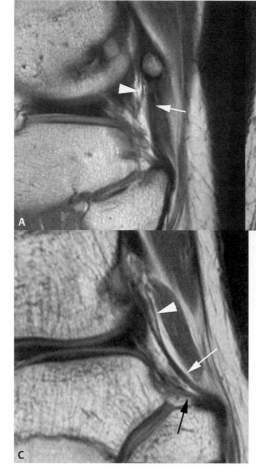

Figure 74–6

to the fibular styloid process with the inferior popliteomeniscal fascicle (PMFi). **Figures 74–5F** to **74–5I** show how the superior popliteomeniscal fascicle (PMF) becomes the meniscocapsular fascicle (MCF) and meniscocapsular junction medial to the popliteus sheath (PS). The fabellofibular ligament (FFL) shares a common posterior attachment to the fibular styloid with the arcuate ligament (AL). The arcuate ligament has a vertically oriented lateral component (ALl) and a more proximal medial component (Alm) that forms the posterior capsular layer of the knee joint deep to the fabellofibular attachment to the fabella (F).

The fabellofibular ligament and its closely allied arcuate ligament are routinely visible on sagittal 3 T images but are rarely resolved at 1.5 T. **Figures 74–6A** and **74–6B** are sagittal proton density and coronal T1 images of particularly prominent fabellofibular ligaments found with routine internal derangement protocol imaging. Arrows indicate the fabellofibular ligaments whereas the arrowhead shows the medial tract of the arcuate ligament. In the absence of a fabella, the fabellofibular ligament fibers appear to get incorporated into the arcuate ligament and posterolateral corner joint capsule, making the arcuate ligament more conspicuous. **Figure 74–6C** is a sagittal proton density image of a skeletally immature girl where the combined fabellofibular-arcuate ligament (white arrow) is well demonstrated in the absence of a fabella. The arrowhead shows the thin divergent fibers of the proximal fabellofibular ligament coursing toward the deep surface of the lateral gastrocnemius. The black arrow shows the popliteofibular ligament.

The popliteus tendon and its meniscal hiatus and posterolateral extension of the knee joint capsule complete the LCL and posterolateral corner complex. Popliteus

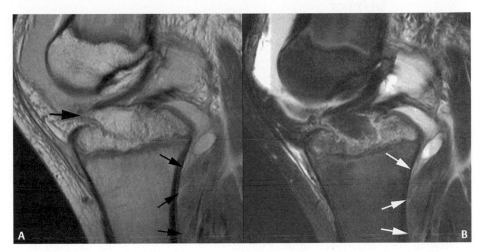

Figure 74–7

muscle strains are far more common than injury to the popliteus tendon and like most posterolateral corner injuries occur with rotational subluxation and ACL tears. **Figures 74–7A** and **74–7B** are sagittal proton density and fat-saturated T2 images of a large avulsion fracture of the intercondylar eminence of the tibia as the result of a violent ACL tug injury. Note the laxity of the anterior band of the ACL as the result of the elevation of its insertion point (large arrow). There is a strain of the popliteus muscle with intrafascicular edema/hemorrhage (small arrows).

75 Wrist

John T. Pitts, Ethan A. Colby, and Jonmenjoy Biswas

Due to its relatively small size and intricate anatomy, the wrist poses significant challenges for imaging. Previously, some of the structures within the wrist that are important for patient management have been difficult to evaluate given the lower SNR inherent at 1.5 T. With the advent of 3 T, the increase in spatial resolution (afforded by improved SNR) has made possible better visualization of anatomy and enhanced lesion detectability.

The triangular fibrocartilage complex (TFCC) is a commonly injured structure of great clinical importance and is well visualized at 3 T. True to its name, the TFCC is composed of a fibrocartilaginous disk and associated ligaments located between the carpus and the ulna. It is analogous to the meniscus in the knee and provides stabilization to the distal radial ulnar joint and the ulnocarpal joint. Laterally, it is attached to the ulnar aspect of the lunate fossa of the radius. **Figure 75–1** presents T1- **(A)** and T2-weighted **(B)** coronal 3 T images with clear visualization of the normal interposition of high signal intensity hyaline cartilage (arrow) between the normal TFCC and its radial attachment. This is not to be mistaken for a tear of the TFCC. On the medial side, two thin bands connect the TFCC to the ulnar styloid. The TFCC inserts distally into the lunate via the ulnolunate ligament and into the triquetrum via the ulnotriquetral ligament.

Like the fibrocartilaginous meniscus of the knee, the TFCC is generally hypointense on all pulse sequences, as demonstrated here. However, it may also display relatively increased intrasubstance signal intensity due to myxoid degeneration. The diagnosis of tear is usually reserved for a high signal intensity abnormality that reaches the surface of the TFCC.

Closely associated with the TFCC is the extensor carpi ulnaris (ECU) tendon, the sheath of which is considered a component of the TFCC. **Figure 75–2** is a comparison

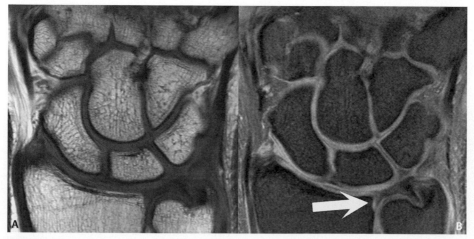

Figure 75–1

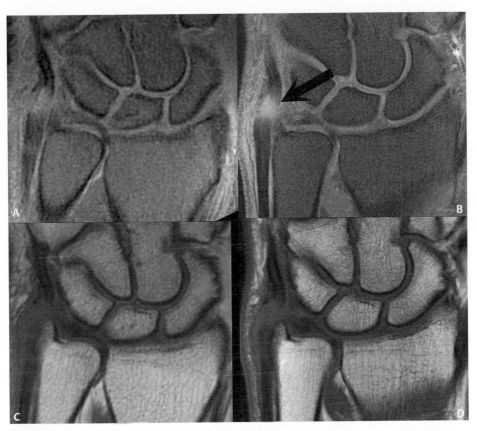

Figure 75–2

of imaging performed at 1.5 T (**Figs. 75–2A** and **75–2C**) and 3 T (**Figs. 75–2B** and **75–2D**) using T1-weighted FSE imaging with and without fat saturation. Note the signal abnormality within the tendon adjacent to the ulnar styloid (arrow). While a normal ECU tendon may exhibit increased signal intensity on T2-weighted images, the degree of signal abnormality and associated thickening of the tendon in the region of the ulnar styloid in this patient is consistent with a partial thickness tear. Fluid signal intensity is also seen to surround the tendon, consistent with the diagnosis of tenosynovitis. SNR measurements on the matched 2-mm T1-weighted coronal images with fat saturation (acquired with identical TR/TE and voxel size) were 24 at 1.5 T (**Fig. 75–2A**) and 47 at 3 T (**Fig. 75–2B**). Scan times were 5:40 (min:sec) at 1.5 T as compared with 3:34 at 3 T.

Figure 75–3 presents paired T2-weighted axial GRE scans demonstrating a ganglion cyst of the radiocarpal joint (black arrow) imaged at 1.5 (**A**) and 3 T (**B**). The scans demonstrate the cyst arising from the volar aspect of the radiocarpal joint in the wrist of this 26-year-old woman, who presented with gradual onset of discomfort and swelling of the right wrist. Ganglion cysts are one of the most common causes of a mass within the wrist and are thought to be the result of chronic irritation at the point of formation. Both scans were acquired with a 2-mm slice thickness, two acquisitions,

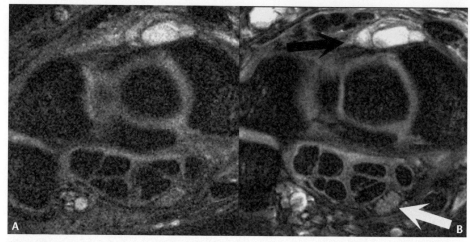

Figure 75–3

a matrix size of 256 × 256, and field of view of 50 × 50. Scan times were 5:02 (min:sec) at 1.5 T and 4:46 at 3 T. In addition to the improved demonstration of the ganglion cyst, note the exquisite detail of the median nerve (white arrow) and the sharp delineation of the tendon sheaths on the 3 T image (due to the markedly higher SNR).

Figure 75–4 presents coronal and sagittal reformatted images from a 3D T2-weighted GRE (dual echo steady state, or DESS) scan of the same lesion, with 0.4 × 0.4 × 0.4 mm^3 resolution. Note the characteristic low signal intensity septations within the cyst that assist in characterization and diagnosis.

The images in **Fig. 75–5** are from the wrist of a 69-year-old man who fell on an out-stretched hand. On history and physical examination, he was found to have dorsal

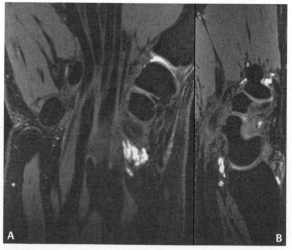

Figure 75–4

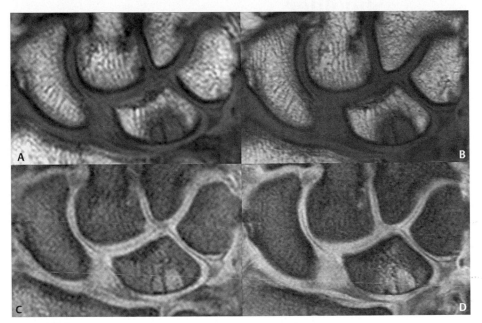

Figure 75–5

pain over the proximal carpus. These images demonstrate an incidentally discovered intraosseous ganglion or subchondral cyst within the lunate. Not so incidental is the widening of the scapholunate distance visualized on these images, consistent with scapholunate instability. This finding was confirmed and repaired during subsequent surgery. **Figures 75–5A** and **75–5C** are T1-weighted coronal images both with **(C)** and without **(A)** fat saturation at 1.5 T. **Figures 75–5B** and **75–5D** are T1-weighted coronal images with **(D)** and without fat saturation **(B)** in same individual at 3 T. The SNR (from region of interest measurements) on the image in **Fig. 75–5C** was 30 at 1.5 T and in the image in **Fig. 75–5D** was 40 at 3 T. Both scans were acquired with a 2-mm slice thickness. In this instance, scan time was reduced from 5:39 (min:sec) at 1.5 T to 3:34 at 3 T. Such a reduction in scan time can be extremely useful clinically when imaging the intricate anatomy of the wrist, where inadvertent patient motion can substantially degrade high-resolution images.

76 Shoulder

Ethan A. Colby and Jonmenjoy Biswas

Of the myriad structures within the shoulder, one of the most difficult to properly image is the labrum. The various types of glenoid labral injuries are legion and may include partial- and full-thickness tears as well as fraying or avulsion of the labrum. Generally, the diagnosis of a labral tear without the use of intra-articular contrast injection is difficult and requires the visualization of linear high signal intensity within the labrum in a characteristic location and orientation. Normal anatomic structures may mimic a labral tear as well.

The high SNR of 3 T can be used to increase spatial resolution allowing for enhanced detection of pathologies of articular cartilage such as labral tears of the shoulder. **Figure 76–1A** is a T2-weighted axial fat-saturated image with an FOV of 170 × 170 mm^2 and voxel dimensions of 0.8 × 0.7 × 3 mm^3. Note the high signal intensity, irregular, linear defect in the posterior labrum (black arrow). This must be differentiated from the normal high signal of hyaline cartilage, which may sometimes undercut the labrum and simulate a tear. In this case, the orientation of the tear is perpendicular to the glenoid and is quite distinct from the normal hyaline cartilage that parallels the surface of the glenoid. Also imaged is a paralabral cyst, a secondary sign of labral tear, seen here closely associated with the injury (white arrow). While the first case was successfully surgically repaired using only routine, noncontrast imaging at 3 T, most labral injuries are best imaged after intra-articular gadolinium chelate contrast injection. **Figure 76–1B** is a postcontrast T1-weighted axial fat-saturated image from a different patient. Note the linear area of high signal intensity contrast seen paralleling the surface of the glenoid. While separation of the anterosuperior labrum from the glenoid is a normal anatomic variant if present anterior to the insertion of the long head of the biceps tendon (large white arrow), this image clearly demonstrates high signal intensity extending posteriorly. This is consistent with the injury

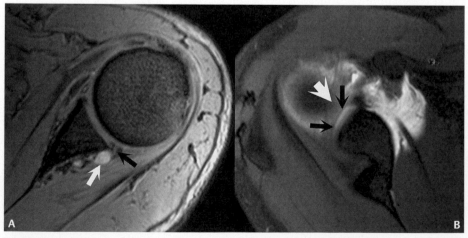

Figure 76–1

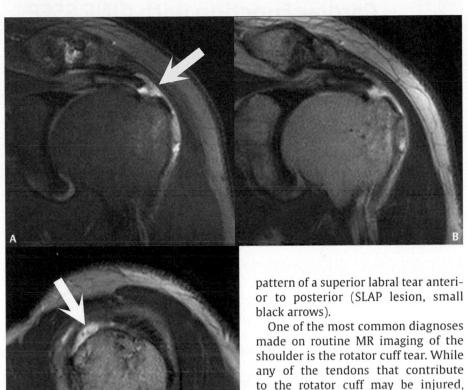

Figure 76–2

pattern of a superior labral tear anterior to posterior (SLAP lesion, small black arrows).

One of the most common diagnoses made on routine MR imaging of the shoulder is the rotator cuff tear. While any of the tendons that contribute to the rotator cuff may be injured, the most commonly affected is the supraspinatus tendon. The patient illustrated in **Fig. 76–2** reported difficulty with overhead activity as well as a decrease in his strength and range of motion. Importantly, 3 T can be used to reduce scan time, which allows for rapid imaging of detailed structures while minimizing the effect of patient motion on image quality. Rapid imaging also minimizes patient discomfort. In addition, parallel imaging can be used to further reduce scan time while maintaining high spatial resolution secondary to the gain in SNR when compared with 1.5 T. **Figure 76–2A** is a T2-weighted coronal sequence (TR/TE = 5790/80) with fat saturation with a scan time of 4:03 (min:sec) using one acquisition and a bandwidth of 180. **Figures 76–2B** and **76–2C** are T2-weighted coronal (TR/TE = 5810/80) and sagittal (TR/TE = 7210/80) scans acquired with one acquisition, a bandwidth of 180, and with scan times of 2:13 and 2:45, respectively. Both of these scans employed a parallel imaging factor of two, reducing scan time in half. The patient had a full-thickness, full-width tear of the supraspinatus tendon (arrow) with 6 mm of tendon retraction. Operative repair was subsequently undertaken with good result.

77 Cardiac Function with CINE SSFP

Bernd J. Wintersperger

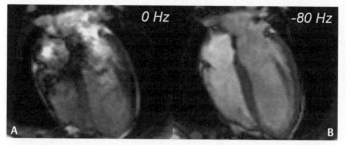

Figure 77–1

The use of steady-state free precession (SSFP) CINE techniques at 3 T is frequently accompanied by imaging artifacts and energy deposition limits. Optimization of SSFP image quality at 3 T requires appropriate scanner and sequence adjustments, which may need to be individualized for each patient. High-quality shimming may eliminate or reduce inhomogeneity and thus artifacts. **Figure 77–1** demonstrates dark band artifacts from off-resonances with additional blood flow–related artifacts. After −80 Hz transmitter frequency shift, artifacts are minimized. Optimization of the transmitter frequency may be facilitated by manually changing the transmitter frequency (steps ~40 Hz; range -200 to 200 Hz) or the use of frequency scouts. **Figure 77–2** shows a series of images at the same position with varying transmitter frequency offsets. The adjustments may be performed best using a four-chamber view to be able to recognize artifacts at various positions within the heart from base to apex. An additional

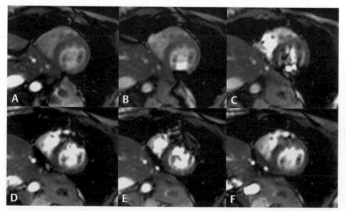

Figure 77–2

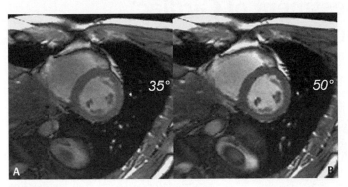

Figure 77–3

view at a midventricular short axis position may add further information in the third dimension. The steady-state nature of these CINE techniques will lead to SAR issues with these sequences at 3 T. Thus lower flip angles may be necessary, resulting in a lower CNR. **Figure 77–3** shows CINE SSFP images acquired at 35 degrees and 50 degrees. Higher flip angles may be possible by using different excitation pulses (slower pulses) though this change sacrifices temporal resolution based on the resulting longer repetition time.

With optimized image quality, CINE SSFP at 3 T allows assessment of global and regional cardiac function and is as accurate as at 1.5 T. An 8-mm slice thickness is still considered the standard, although the improved SNR at 3 T will likely allow for thinner sections of 4 to 6 mm while maintaining high image quality. If thinner slices are to be used, care needs to be taken to provide sufficient coverage of the ventricles using interslice gaps of not more than 2 mm. In-plane spatial resolution is typically in the range of 1.4 to 2.0 mm with a temporal resolution of <50 msec (typically ~30 to 45 msec). Data acquisition is in the range of 7 to 9 heartbeats per slice. Parallel imaging algorithms allow substantially faster data acquisition at the cost of SNR. **Figure 77–4** shows a whole short axis CINE data set acquired in two breath-holds of 15 heartbeats each with fourfold acceleration using TSENSE.

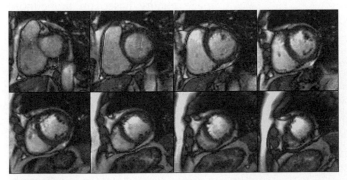

Figure 77–4

78 Assessment of Cardiac Morphology

Bernd J. Wintersperger

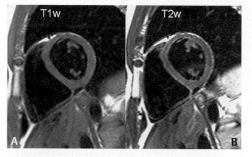

Figure 78–1

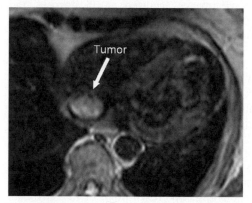

Figure 78–2

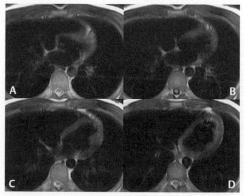

Figure 78–3

Morphologic MR imaging techniques are commonly used for assessment of congenital heart disease (CHD) or acquired diseases such as a cardiac mass. The imaging technique employed is strongly dependent on the reason for imaging referral. Most often, single-slice turbo spin-echo (TSE) techniques or its multislice derivatives are applied. These techniques include black-blood preparation to null signal of the cavitary blood pool and thus enable artifact-free images. **Figure 78–1** shows comparative short axis slices of a T1-weighted and a T2-weighted TSE sequence.

At 3 T, TSE technique may be limited by the SAR, thus flip angles need to be reduced or specific low SAR pulses used. In addition, although not specific to any field strength, effective TR values depend on the patient's RR interval and may only be as short as a single RR interval. **Figure 78–2** shows an axial T2-weighted TSE slice with an effective TR of 3 heartbeats, leading to the markedly high signal of the metastasis (arrow) within the right atrium from advanced adrenal carcinoma. At 3 T, surrounding lung tissue may impair image quality based on pronounced susceptibility artifacts. This is especially common in half-Fourier acquisition single-shot turbo-spine echo (HASTE) imaging, a technique commonly used for accelerated T2-weighted imaging at 1.5 T. **Figure 78–3** shows multiple axial slices acquired with a HASTE technique at 3 T that demonstrates this problem, with the free right ventricular wall hardly visible.

T1-weighted techniques are required to assess contrast uptake in inflammation and within cardiac masses. After

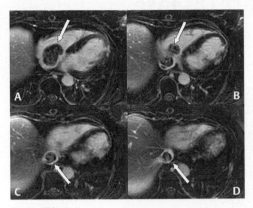

Figure 78–4

contrast application though, artifact-free images of the blood pool may not be achievable. Inversion recovery GRE techniques, as used also in delayed enhancement imaging, can alternatively be employed for tumor detection and delineation. **Figure 78–4** demonstrates the same right atrial tumor (arrows) as presented in **Fig. 78–2** with excellent delineation of the blood pool and the wall in addition to the inhomogeneous lesion enhancement. In almost any morphologic cardiac MR referral, the use of dynamic imaging techniques such as CINE SSFP provides added value. In CHD, shunt volumes may be quantified by assessment of the right and left ventricular function or hemodynamic alterations (e.g., stenosis) shown by flow turbulence. In mass assessment, the possible impact on cardiac function may also be detected. **Figure 78–5** shows the same tumor thrombus as in **Fig. 78–4** imaged with a CINE SSFP technique. The tumor prolapses into the tricuspid valve annulus during diastolic filling.

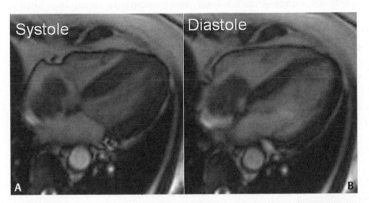

Figure 78–5

79 Ischemic Heart Disease

Bernd J. Wintersperger

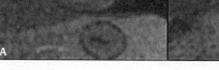

Figure 79–1

Coronary artery disease (CAD) and its sequelae are among the major causes of mortality in Western countries. MR imaging at 1.5 T has been shown to be of substantial value in diagnosis of CAD in recent years. Flow-limiting coronary stenosis may be identified using perfusion imaging during pharmacologic stress conditions and at rest. Typically, MR myocardial perfusion imaging is based on magnetization prepared fast GRE techniques (e.g., saturation recovery TurboFLASH) that image each individual slice at every heartbeat. This high temporal resolution is mandatory to allow for adequate assessment of contrast agent kinetics during inflow of an extracellular gadolinium-based contrast agent. **Figure 79–1** shows two slices depicting a large myocardial perfusion deficit (arrows) acquired at 1.5 T. The patient has a known history of extensive anterior myocardial infarction. Imaging is performed with an 8-mm slice thickness and a 192 matrix size. **Figure 79–2** shows the same patient during perfusion

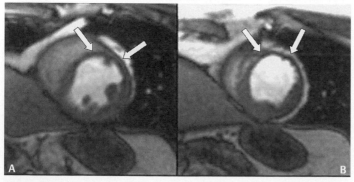

Figure 79–2

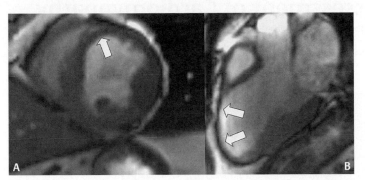

Figure 79–3

assessment at 3 T. Due to the increase in field strength, there is substantially improved SNR. The higher SNR enables a better visual delineation of perfusion abnormalities (arrows) as well as a more accurate time-intensity analysis. In assessment of coronary artery stenosis, myocardial perfusion imaging is usually performed at rest and during pharmacologic stress. This allows for an evaluation of the myocardial perfusion reserve. Besides the assessment of myocardial perfusion, the workup of CAD consists of CINE imaging of the heart and viability assessment. **Figure 79–3** demonstrates substantial anterior wall thinning (arrows) without systolic thickening in the same patient as shown in the perfusion images. Using delayed enhancement techniques with IR TurboFLASH after double dose injection of a standard gadolinium chelate, the infarcted area lights up with proper TI settings in an image data set acquired ~10 min after injection. In a combined setting of perfusion imaging and delayed enhancement techniques, residual contrast from perfusion studies is still present, thus the injection of an additional single dose after the perfusion study may be sufficient. **Figure 79–4** demonstrates the extensive transmural delayed enhancement (arrows) in the anterior wall matching the myocardial thinning as shown in perfusion and CINE imaging. This enhanced area reflects nonviable myocardium with extensive scar tissue. In the case of acute myocardial infarction, delayed enhancing areas represent necrotic myocardial tissue with increased contrast agent distribution volume based on interstitial edema and ruptured cell membranes.

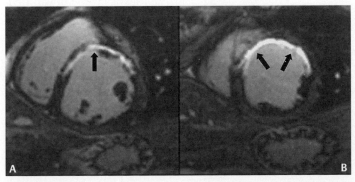

Figure 79–4

80 Assessment of Cardiomyopathy

Bernd J. Wintersperger

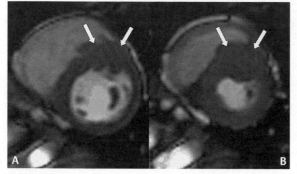

Figure 80–1

Cardiomyopathies represent a heterogeneous group of various diseases that are of either primary or secondary origin. The most common secondary cardiomyopathies include ischemic cardiomyopathy with ventricular dilation and hypertrophic cardiomyopathy based on long-standing arterial hypertension or aortic stenosis. Primary cardiomyopathies originally did not have any known underlying disease, but detailed research work has gradually revealed new insights into these disorders. MR imaging has been shown to contribute to the diagnosis of primary and secondary cardiomyopathy mainly based on the use of dynamic imaging capabilities (e.g., function) and the concept of "delayed enhancement" imaging. **Figure 80–1** shows a basal short axis slice in systole and diastole in a 24-year-old patient with hypertrophic cardiomyopathy and suspicion of left ventricular outflow tract obstruction. The myocardium is primarily thickened in the anteroseptal region (arrows) while the lateral and inferior wall segments are normal. **Figure 80–2** shows the outflow tract in a three-chamber view. Although the septum is markedly thickened, the outflow tract is not obstructed during systole. Also, there is no sign of anterior mitral

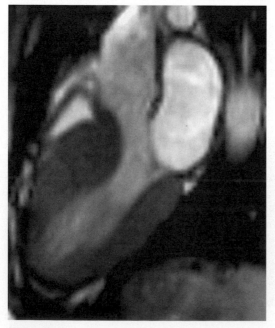

Figure 80–2

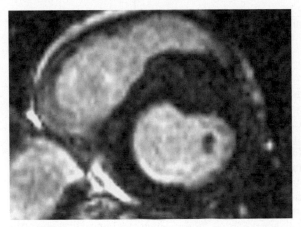

Figure 80–3

valve leaflet doming that additionally may narrow the outflow tract.

Cardiomyopathies may be accompanied by myocardial fibrosis in addition to a disarray of the myocardial fibers. Changes of the composition of the ventricular wall will result in changed properties of the extracellular space. Hence, these changes will be visible using "delayed enhancement" T1-weighted techniques. The concept of delayed enhancement has been extensively studied at 1.5 T. The use of a higher field strength (i.e., 3 T) will result in a higher contrast-to-noise ratio (CNR) of abnormal myocardial areas and thus allow better depiction of subtle changes. Whereas at 1.5 T inversion recovery (IR) SSFP sequence techniques have been proposed based on superior CNR, at 3 T these techniques encounter the same artifact problems as CINE SSFP imaging (see Case 77). The preferred approach for delayed enhancement imaging at 3 T is the use of IR TurboFLASH sequence techniques with a slice thickness of 6 to 8 mm. Due to the prolonged T1 values at 3 T, the best inversion time (TI) is typically longer than at 1.5 T and should be optimized using techniques that automatically acquire images at various TI (TI scouts). Based on these techniques, the optimal TI can be chosen. **Figure 80–3**, a delayed enhancement image in the patient also presented in **Figs. 80–1** and **80–2**, does not show any evidence of abnormal contrast enhancement and thus indicates the absence of myocardial fibrosis. **Figure 80–4** shows an IR TurboFLASH image in long axis orientation in a patient with severe apical hypertrophic cardiomyopathy, with abnormal contrast enhancement (arrows) indicating extensive fibrosis in that area.

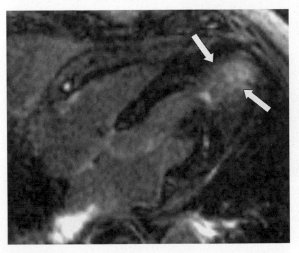

Figure 80–4

81 Breast
Mitchell D. Schnall

MR breast imaging has gained widespread clinical acceptance for applications extending from high-risk screening to cancer evaluation and therapy response. By using architecture/morphologic criteria, contrast kinetics, and newer approaches such as intensity-modulated parametric mapping technique, better distinction between benign and malignant disease can be achieved. With the advent of 3 T, and accompanying improved spatial and temporal resolution capabilities, breast MR clinical applications can be substantially enhanced. **Figure 81–1A** demonstrates a single sagittal slice from a bilateral dynamic breast MR imaging exam that acquired 32 slices from each breast as two concurrently acquired slabs using a 384 × 192 matrix (TR = 8.2 msec, TE = 3.2 msec, FOV = 18 cm, slice thickness = 3 mm, flip angle = 15 degrees, with spectral fat suppression). This image is the first postcontrast image from a dynamic postcontrast acquisition that acquired images over 7 min. The acquisition time was 45 sec for each image set. **Fig. 81–1A** demonstrates rapid prominent enhancement of an invasive breast cancer that was detected by clinical exam and difficult to detect on mammography **(Fig. 81–1B)**. MR imaging has been demonstrated to be of high utility for the detection and characterization of

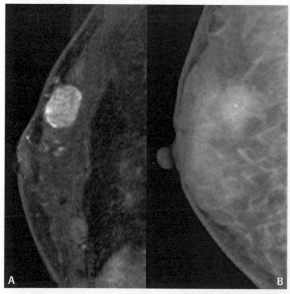

Figure 81–1

breast cancer based on the use of dynamic contrast enhanced scans. Although most of the information regarding MR imaging performance is based on data at 1.5 T, there is strong reason to believe that the performance at 3 T will be better. There are several factors that lead us to this assessment, one factor being the size of the breast, which allows efficient coils to be designed for 3 T. Additionally, the breast tends to have a large fatty content, which reduces the effect of the tissue loading on the coil performance, resulting in highly efficient RF coils that are poised to reap much of the theoretical signal-to-noise advantage of 3 T. Another factor is that the key scan type tends to be a 3D GRE acquisition with a small flip angle, which reduces the impact of the increased SAR associated with 3 T (SAR being proportional to the square of the flip angle amplitude). Also, the increased tissue T1 times for glandular tissue at 3 T associated with the improved effectiveness of the standard gadolinium chelates at 3 T compared with that at 1.5 T (see Case 27) combine to give higher contrast between enhancing and nonenhancing background tissue. Lastly, an increase in the chemical shift dispersion (frequency difference between species with different chemical shifts) improves the effectiveness of fat suppression and reduces the time required to play out spectrally selective pulses by a factor of two, reducing the impact of fat suppression on scan time.

Figures 81–2A and **81–2B** compares images obtained with parameters similar to that described above at 1.5 T **(A)** and 3 T **(B)**. These images represent subtraction images from the first postcontrast acquisition of a dynamic series and illustrate a large breast carcinoma. Note the increased SNR in the 3 T scan relative to the 1.5 T

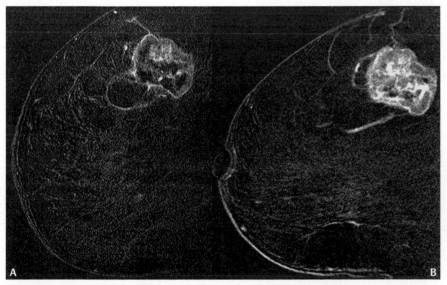

Figure 81–2

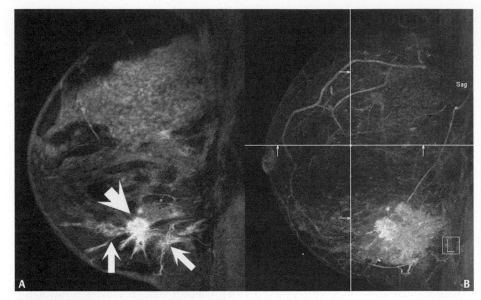

Figure 81–3

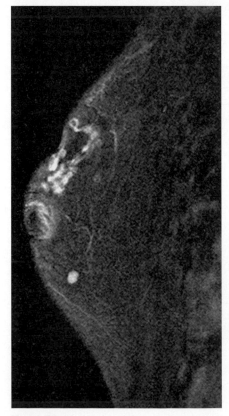

Figure 81–4

scan. These data illustrate that the SNR advantages at 3 T are real. We have found ~1.7 times the SNR for 3 T imaging of the breast relative to 1.5 T using similar acquisition parameters. The increase in SNR and more efficient fat suppression at 3 T can be leveraged to improve image resolution, as well as to improve time or spatial resolution of the dynamic postcontrast acquisition. An example of increasing the spatial resolution is demonstrated in **Fig. 81–3A**. What this image represents is a single sagittal slice from a bilateral dynamic breast MR imaging exam that acquired 32 slices from each breast as two concurrently acquired slabs using an 896 × 448 matrix (TR = 8.9 msec, TE = 3.7 msec, FOV = 18 cm, slice thickness = 3 mm, flip angle = 15 degrees, with spectral fat suppression). The total acquisition time was 120 sec. The in-plane image resolution is 0.2×0.4 mm^2. The primary invasive cancer (large arrow) and associated intraductal extent (small arrows) are clearly visible. **Figure 81–3B** presents a 3D MIP reconstruction showing the full extent of the lesion.

Improved resolution with 3 T, by minimizing volume averaging with smaller voxel sizes, thus providing higher tissue contrast, allows for substantially improved identification of infiltrating disease not appreciated on conventional imaging modalities, better delineation of lesions, and a reduction in re-excision rates. **Figure 81–4** illustrates a high-resolution dynamic postcontrast image acquired with the protocol described above. The individual ducts that compose this patient's ductal carcinoma in situ (DCIS) are visualized. Although there is not enough clinical experience with 3 T to date, it is hoped that 3 T will allow more effective detection of DCIS, a known weakness of 1.5 T MRI.

82 Liver: Spatial Resolution

Christoph J. Zech

Due to advanced therapeutic possibilities for focal liver disease including specialized surgery and minimally invasive approaches (e.g., radio-frequency ablation and selective internal radiation therapy), accurate staging of hepatic disease is necessary for assigning patients to the most appropriate therapy. Even very subtle imaging findings can be critical to note and interpret correctly for proper patient management.

Modern multidetector computed tomography (MDCT) provides very high spatial resolution with sub-millimeter collimation. However, the reconstructed slice thickness cannot be lower than ~3 mm due to the poor SNR with smaller voxel sizes. This is of particular relevance for liver imaging because many lesions have only low or intermediate contrast on CT, relative to the surrounding liver parenchyma, and may not be detected when too much image noise is present. In this light, MR imaging of the liver at high field is of particular interest, because the higher magnetic field strength results in increased SNR. With modern 1.5 T systems utilizing parallel imaging, a slice thickness of 3 to 4 mm is already possible within a single breath-hold, when 3D GRE sequences with low flip angles are chosen. The use of these 3D GRE sequences appears particularly promising at 3 T, because a further increase in spatial resolution (specifically a further reduction in slice thickness) would be feasible.

Figures 82–1A to **82–1E** show the influence of the slice thickness on image quality in an unenhanced T1-weighted 3D GRE sequence at 3 T. The images are from a 26-year-old female volunteer, with a small liver cyst

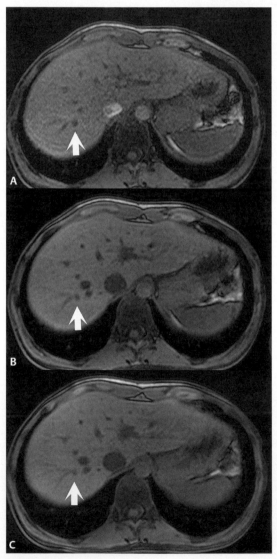

Figure 82–1

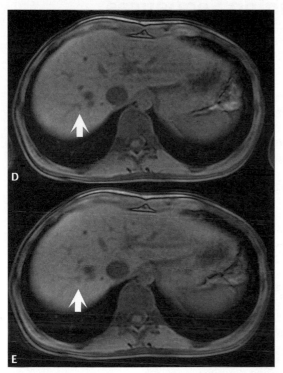

Figure 82–1 *(Continued)*

(arrow) incidentally noted and the focus of subsequent discussion. Slice thicknesses in 1-mm increments are illustrated from **(A)** 1 to **(E)** 5 mm using the same unenhanced T1-weighted sequence. All other sequence parameters were held constant, with an in-plane matrix of 320 × 260 mm², an FOV of 380 × 320 mm², TR = 4.36 msec, TE = 1.59 msec, flip angle = 15 degrees, bandwidth of 300 Hz/pixel, parallel imaging with GRAPPA reconstruction $R = 2$, and a 17-sec breath-hold. The tiny cyst (arrow) is best visualized with a slice thickness of 2 mm, which is also the slice thickness for our routine liver imaging protocol at 3 T. With a slice thickness of 1 mm, image noise becomes dominant, possibly obscuring low-contrast lesions. From 3 mm on, partial volume effects are visible, which lower the contrast of the lesion relative to the surrounding liver parenchyma substantially. With a slice thickness of 5 mm, as shown in **Fig. 82–1E**, the tiny cyst is poorly visualized due to the indistinct (blurred) margins and low contrast, on the basis of partial volume imaging due to the relatively thick section.

For liver imaging at 3 T, T1-weighted 3D GRE sequences can be acquired with a thinner slice thickness as compared with the optimal reconstructed slice thickness in MDCT, which has been proposed to be between 3 and 5 mm. In comparison of the two modalities, this favors 3 T MR, with potential advantages for detection of small and ultrasmall lesions.

83 Liver: Imaging Sequences

Christoph J. Zech

Despite the obvious advantages of high-field MR, several drawbacks have limited early use of 3 T systems for abdominal imaging, in addition to other reasons. In particular, dielectric artifacts can cause severe problems especially on T2-weighted sequences, fat suppression is considered not as robust as on 1.5 T systems in the abdomen, and SAR constraints have to be considered.

Figures 83–1A to **83–1D** demonstrate that MR imaging of the liver at 3 T is feasible with good image quality using the standard T1- and T2-weighted fast sequences that are deemed necessary for liver imaging. The case presents images from the exam of a 64-year-old male patient with a history of rectal carcinoma. An ultrasound examination performed for hepatic staging questioned a lesion in the right lobe of the liver, of uncertain etiology, and the patient was referred to MR imaging, which was performed on a 3 T system.

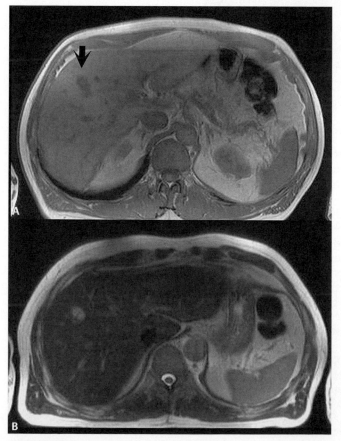

Figure 83–1

Imaging consisted of a T1-weighted 2D in-phase GRE sequence **(A)**, a T2-weighted single shot sequence (HASTE) **(B)**, and postcontrast 3D GRE scans with fat saturation at 20 **(C)** and 50 sec **(D)** after injection of an extracellular gadolinium chelate. All scans demonstrate good to excellent image quality. The lesion in question (arrow) is hypointense on the T1-weighted scan precontrast and moderately hyperintense on the T2-weighted scan. After contrast injection, the lesion demonstrates rim-enhancement and fast washout, with the center of the lesion remaining low signal intensity (hypovascularized). The imaging characteristics are consistent with a colorectal carcinoma metastasis to the liver, which was confirmed by surgical resection.

Note the slight signal nonuniformities across the FOV in all scans, which correspond with B_1-inhomogenities. This phenomenon is well-known in abdominal high-field MR imaging; however, in our opinion and consistent with early study results by our group, this does not interfere with image interpretation. The spatial resolution of the exam is high with a 5-mm slice thickness employed for the 2D sequences **(A, B)** and a 2-mm slice thickness for the 3D sequences **(C, D)**. The in-plane matrix was 384×256 mm^2 for **(A)**, 320×256 mm^2 for **(B)**, and 320×192 mm^2 for **(C)** and **(D)** with a FOV of 350×300 mm^2 for all sequences. Fat-suppression is uniform, as applied on the contrast enhanced scans. There were no problems with regard to SAR limits in this patient, which has also been our experience in the majority of patient exams.

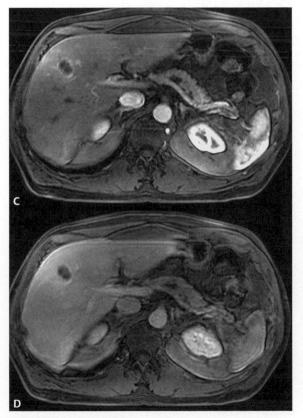

Figure 83–1 *(Continued)*

84 Liver: Ultra-small Metastases

Christoph J. Zech

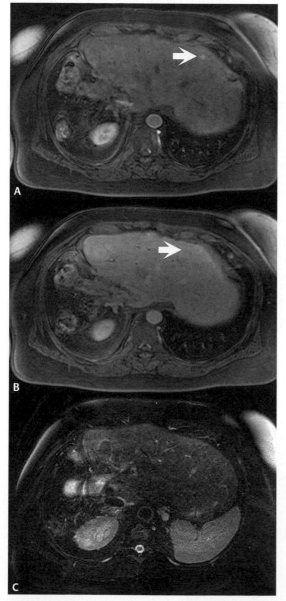

Figure 84–1

As pointed out in Case 82, the challenge for liver MR imaging is to detect ultra-small liver metastases. The combination of favorable SNR at high field and liver-specific contrast agents (which provide increased contrast between liver metastases and the surrounding parenchyma) leads to a synergistic effect that makes possible high-resolution scans with excellent lesion contrast. Examples of liver-specific gadolinium chelates include gadobenate dimeglumine (Gd BOPTA, or MultiHance, Bracco Diagnostics, Princeton, NJ, USA) and gadoxetic acid (Gd EOB-DTPA, or Primovist, Schering AG, Berlin, Germany). The former is approved worldwide for clinical use, with the latter approved in Europe since 2004 and marketing authorization still pending in the United States.

Figures 84–1A to **84–1E** present MR images at both 1.5 and 3 T of a 49-year-old female patient suffering from a Klatskin tumor (this was a follow-up exam after resection). **Figures 84–1A** and **84–1B** present early dynamic images after bolus injection of Primovist, specifically in the arterial and portal venous phases. The arrow points to a tiny hypervascular subcapsular metastasis. As would be expected with a conventional extracellular contrast agent, this small hypervascular lesion demonstrates early enhancement in the arterial phase, with

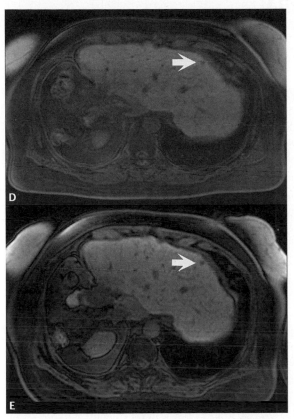

Figure 84–1 *(Continued)*

subsequent washout in the portal venous phase. In the latter instance (**B**), the lesion cannot be detected due to its isointensity in this phase with surrounding normal liver.

The first part of the exam was performed on a 1.5 T magnet with a T1-weighted 3D GRE sequence using a 3-mm slice thickness. **Figure 84–1C** presents the respiratory triggered, T2-weighted, fat-suppressed FSE scan from the first part of the exam, on which the lesion cannot be detected due to its relative isointensity to normal liver. Thus a small high-flow hemangioma (Semelka type 1) can be ruled out. Such a lesion would be depicted with high signal intensity on the T2-weighted scan. At ~20 min after injection, imaging in the hepatocyte-specific phase with Primovist can be initiated. **Figure 84–1D** shows the liver-specific phase of the 1.5 T exam. Immediately after this scan, a 2-mm T1-weighted 3D GRE sequence (**E**) was performed on the 3 T system. In the hepatocyte phase of Primovist, a hypervascular metastasis should be hypointense (due to the absence of normal hepatocytes), as with all other metastases. Looking at the exam overall, the lesion can be diagnosed with high confidence as a metastasis because of the washout of contrast from the lesion on the one hand (during dynamic imaging) and the lack of enhancement during the liver-specific delayed phase on the other hand, despite its small size. Although the image quality and depiction of these subtle findings are good on the 1.5 T scans, 3 T (**E**) provides a further improvement in lesion contrast and definition of the margin of the lesion, due to reduced partial volume imaging.

85 Liver: SPIO

Christoph J. Zech

Imaging of the cirrhotic liver is a challenging issue in abdominal MR imaging. Because of the presence of diffuse alterations in the liver parenchyma, the poor state of health of the patients, and the presence of ascites, acceptable image quality and proper assessment of pathologies can be difficult to achieve. This holds especially true for

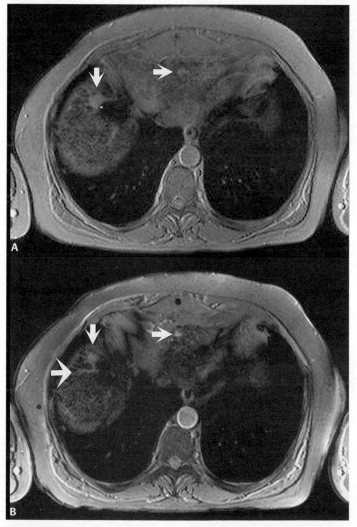

Figure 85–1

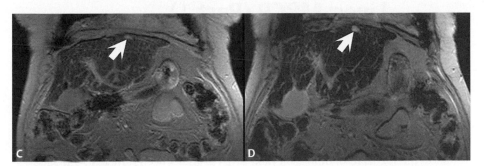

Figure 85–1 *(Continued)*

imaging at 3 T, where ascites can be the reason for pronounced dielectric artifacts, according to preliminary reports in the literature. Presented in **Figs. 85–1A** to **85–1D** are axial and coronal T2*-weighted GRE scans acquired 10 min after bolus injection of the superparamagnetic iron oxide (SPIO) particle ferucarbotran (Resovist, Schering AG, Berlin, Germany) at 1.5 T (**Figs. 85–1A** and **85–1C**) and 3 T (**Figs. 85–1B** and **85–1D**). For both exams, multichannel MR systems were used (Magnetom Avanto and Magnetom Tim Trio, Siemens Medical Solutions, Erlangen, Germany). Parameters for the axial sequence at 1.5 T included a 6-mm slice thickness (10% gap), 256 × 256 matrix, and four image stacks each acquired during a breath-hold of 18 sec. The corresponding parameters for 3 T were 5-mm slice thickness (10% gap), 320 × 256 matrix, and four stacks each acquired during a breath-hold of 17 sec. The FOV was 380 × 320 mm² for both exams.

The basic principle for SPIO imaging is that the signal loss in T2*-weighted sequences indicates uptake of iron particles in the Kupffer cells of the liver, which is the expected finding for normal liver parenchyma. It is known that in cirrhotic or fibrotic livers a reticular, diffuse decrease in SPIO uptake can be seen. In this respect, high-field MR may be of value due to the higher sensitivity to susceptibility (T2*) effects, which is illustrated in this patient exam. Specifically, the liver parenchyma appears more hypointense ("darker") on the 3 T scans. This provides greater contrast, relative to adjacent normal liver, for the nodules completely lacking iron uptake. These can be identified in liver segments 2 and 8 (arrows) and correspond with small hepatocellular carcinoma nodules. Note also the excellent depiction of fibrosis (as linear streaks) in the liver at 3 T (large arrow), facilitating the differentiation between nodular tumor and areas of fibrosis. This problem arises commonly in daily clinical practice in the cirrhotic patient population.

Although the patient presented here had some ascites, no problems with dielectric artifacts were noted in this case. However, based on personal experience, ascites can be problematic in regard to both motion artifacts and dielectric artifacts.

86 Liver: MRCP (Part 1)

Christoph J. Zech

Magnetic resonance cholangiopancreatography (MRCP) is accepted as the noninvasive standard for assessment of biliary pathologies. With MRCP, biliary obstruction, cholelithiasis, and malignant strictures can be diagnosed with high confidence. However, for biliary disease with only subtle changes of the biliary duct caliber, in some instances the spatial resolution achievable at 1.5 T has not been sufficient. One such disease entity is primary sclerosing cholangitis (PSC). In the initial phase of the disease, often only subtle changes in the second- and third-order biliary branches can be seen, with dilatations and small stenoses ("string of beads"). For these patients, the improvement in spatial resolution that can be gained at 3 T is expected to be beneficial. This hypothesis has been confirmed in our preliminary experience.

Figure 86–1 presents images from a T2-weighted 3D FSE scan acquired at 3 T with an isotropic 0.9 mm³ voxel size. Time of acquisition for such a data set is usually between 3 and 5 min with respiratory triggering (using a respiratory belt or navigator techniques such as prospective acquisition correction [PACE]) when parallel imaging with an acceleration factor of $R = 2$ is used. **(A)** and **(B)** are consecutive thin MIPs, which show two involved biliary ducts (arrows, draining segment 5/6). **Figures 86–1C**

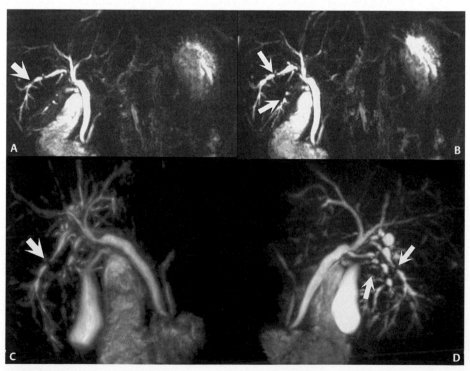

Figure 86–1

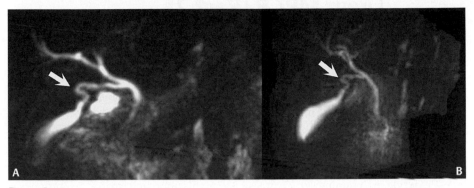

Figure 86–2

and **86–1D** present volume rendering of the acquired data set with a view from anterior **(C)** and posterior **(D)**. Such postprocessing gives a fast and realistic overview of the anatomy together with localization of pathology and can be helpful for demonstration of findings to referring and consulting physicians (e.g., the endoscopist). **Figures 86–2A** and **86–2B** show the biliary system of a healthy volunteer with the same high-resolution T2-weighted 3D FSE sequence. In this example, no biliary congestion is present. Note the excellent depiction of the cystic duct (arrow) in **Fig. 86–2A** (a thin MIP). **Figure 86–2B** (a thick MIP) again provides an overview of the entire biliary system, showing absence of pathologic findings.

Figures 86–3A and **86–3B** show the comparison of a RARE (rapid acquisition with relaxation enhancement) sequence, used for thick-slab MRCP, acquired at 1.5 T **(A)** and 3 T **(B)** in 47-year-old female patient. The slab thickness was 50 mm for both scans, with an acceleration factor of $R = 3$ used in each case. The in-plane resolution was 384×320 at 1.5 T and 448×448 at 3 T with an identical FOV (350×350 mm^2). TR and TE were 4500 and 754 msec, respectively. The exam is normal, without pathologic findings. Note the artifact involving the common bile duct (signal extinction) due to flow within the hepatic artery (arrow), visible at both field strengths. The superior SNR and spatial resolution at 3 T result in better contrast of the biliary system relative to the background, with increased visualization of both the peripheral biliary tree as well as the pancreatic duct (small arrows). The time interval between the two exams was 24 hours, with the patient not fasting prior to the exam at 3 T.

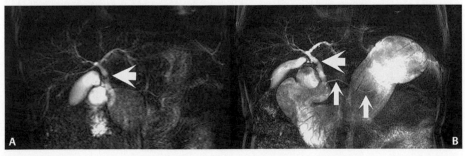

Figure 86–3

87 Liver: MRCP (Part 2)

Elmar M. Merkle

MRCP has become even more clinically useful since the development of respiratory-triggered 3D T2-weighted FSE techniques. These sequences allow for nearly isotropic voxel data sets, with a spatial resolution in the range of 1 mm³. One problem with this approach, however, despite the excellent spatial resolution, is the long acquisition times (TA). New sequence designs such as SPACE (sampling perfection with application of optimized contrasts using different flip angle evolutions) reduce the TA by ~25% while maintaining sufficient SNR. With this approach, spatial resolution can be further improved reaching voxel sizes below 1 mm³. Image quality is also substantially improved by the elimination of N/2 ghost artifacts and improved suppression of the liver background signal. A standard FSE T2-weighted sequence with a fixed refocusing flip angle is only able to acquire half of the k-space lines per partition in a single respiratory cycle. If there are any differences in the diaphragm position between the two halves of k-space, then characteristic N/2 ghost artifacts may appear. Because the SPACE sequence acquires an entire k-space partition in a single respiratory cycle, N/2 ghost artifacts are completely eliminated. In **Fig. 87–1, (A)** was acquired in 4:57 min:sec with a fixed refocusing flip angle of 136 degrees using conventional 3D T2-weighed FSE, producing however insufficient suppression of the liver background signal; **(B)** was acquired in 3:53 min:sec using SPACE with a parallel imaging factor of three and variable refocusing flip angles between 120 degrees and 90 degrees. The latter image shows excellent liver background suppression while maintaining sufficient SNR for diagnostic purposes. **Figure 87–1B** provides improved delineation of the right hepatic duct (large arrow), which is unremarkable in this patient. Note that the implementation of parallel imaging in combination with variable refocusing pulses preserves adequate SNR to permit visualization of nondilated fourth-order biliary branches (small arrow). Incidentally seen in this clinical case are multiple simple liver cysts. A minor drawback of MRCP at 3 T currently is the presence of dielectric artifacts in ~15% of cases.

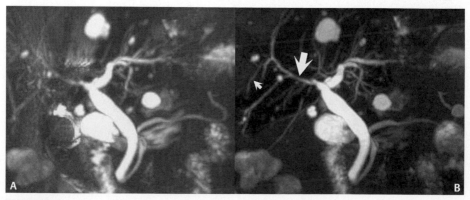

Figure 87–1

88 Kidney (Part 1)

Elizabeth M. Hecht and Benjamin Hyman

The Bosniak classification is broadly accepted as a reference for distinguishing between complex renal cysts and cystic renal tumors. Class I/II/IIF lesions are nonoperative/benign lesions, whereas class III/IV are lesions with malignant characteristics that require surgical treatment and pathologic correlation. Shortcomings within the classification have been in accurately distinguishing between class II/IIF and class III lesions by CT or ultrasound. Fortunately, early studies of 3 T versus 1.5 T MR of the abdomen have shown qualitative and quantitatively improved image quality at 3 T, which could lead to better characterization of complex cystic renal lesions. Specific gains are seen with the ability of achieving smaller fields of view, improved in-plane spatial resolution, and thinner slices without sacrificing image quality. In addition to the increased SNR with 3 T, there is significantly higher CNR after gadolinium chelate administration as compared with 1.5 T, improving substantially soft tissue delineation and lesion enhancement (see Case 27).

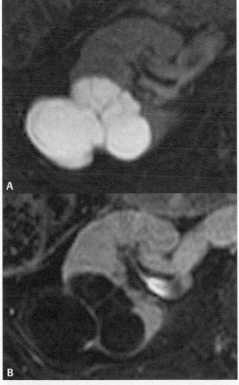

Figures **88–1A** and **88–1B** demonstrate at 3 T axial FSE T2-weighted and postcontrast T1-weighted VIBE scans of a class IIF Bosniak lesion of the right kidney with multiple hairline septa and minimal wall thickening. No distinct enhancing soft tissue elements can be seen on the postcontrast study defining the class of this lesion **(B)**. Further studies and improvements are needed to resolve issues with B_1 field inhomogeneity, motion artifact, and chemical shift seen with high-field MR imaging of the body. However, better characterization of benign and malignant renal cystic lesions with 3 T appears achievable and stands to improve our discriminatory capabilities of these lesions.

Figure 88–1

89 Kidney (Part 2)
Elmar M. Merkle

The adequate staging of renal cell cancer is of utmost importance for successful treatment planning and optimal patient outcome. Staging includes assessment of the renal capsule, perinephric fat and Gerota's fascia; careful search for tumor extension into the renal vein, inferior vena cava and/or regional lymph nodes; and the assessment of direct tumor extension into neighboring structures and search for distant metastases. Contrast-enhanced MR imaging has the capability to answer all these key questions without the burden of nephrotoxicity. At 3 T, FSE-based T2-weighted imaging such as HASTE (**Fig. 89–1A**) permits detection of a clear-cell renal cell cancer and preliminary staging with assessment of the regional lymph nodes and the inferior vena cava. Unenhanced 3D GRE T1-weighted imaging such as VIBE (**Fig. 89–1C**) also allows detection of the primary tumor and enlarged para-aortic lymph nodes but does not permit adequate assessment of vascular involvement. Multiplanar VIBE imaging (**Fig. 89–1B**, axial, and **Fig. 89–1D**, coronal) after administration of a gadolinium chelate provides excellent visualization of the primary tumor, which involves the whole left kidney, with adequate assessment of the left renal vein (small white arrows, **Fig. 89–1B**) and the inferior vena cava, which are free of tumor. In addition, enlarged para-aortic lymph nodes are identified (asterisks in **Fig. 89–1D**). Also note the profound enhancement of Gerota's fascia indicative of parasitizing vessels as well as the irregular appearance of Gerota's fascia itself (small black arrows, **D**). Both findings suggest extension of the tumor beyond the layer of Gerota's fascia.

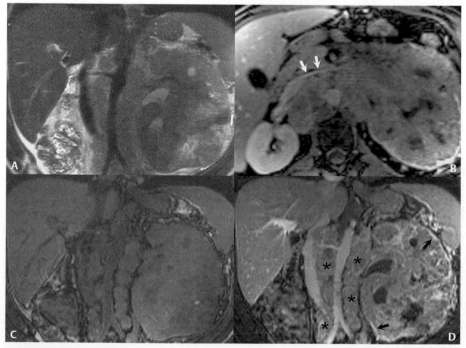

Figure 89–1

90   Kidney: Arterial Spin-Labeling

Andreas Boss, Petros Martirosian, and Fritz Schick

Renal perfusion measurements can provide important diagnostic information in patients with renal artery stenosis, inflammatory and degenerative kidney disease, and renal tumors. Perfusion measurements are usually performed in clinical practice using contrast-enhanced T1-weighted imaging, which requires the intravenous injection of a gadolinium chelate. An alternative approach is a technique termed *arterial spin-labeling* (ASL), in which magnetically labeled blood is used as an endogenous tracer (see Case 54). In the pulsed ASL approach, two images of the same slice with different spin preparations are recorded. For example, in the FAIR (flow-sensitive alternating inversion recovery) scheme, one image with a slice-selective inversion pre-pulse and one image with global inversion are acquired. A perfusion-weighted image can then be generated by subtraction of the two images, with the difference in magnetization proportional to tissue perfusion.

ASL at 3 T provides distinctly higher image quality when compared with 1.5 T because of two different effects. First, MR imaging at 3 T doubles the potential available SNR when compared with 1.5 T. As the perfusion-related magnetization difference is related to the tissue equilibrium magnetization, the perfusion-related signal yield doubles at 3 T as well. A further advantage at 3 T for ASL derives from the longer T1 relaxation time of blood (~20%), leading to an additional increase in perfusion-related signal yield.

Because susceptibility effects scale with field strength, a suitable readout technique needs to be chosen for 3 T. Echoplanar imaging (EPI) strategies, which are conventionally applied for ASL data acquisition at 1.5 T, show strong distortions and signal dephasing in areas of high susceptibility differences, such as the abdomen. Single-shot FSE approaches suffer from significant blurring, which is caused by the faster decay of the echo train at higher field strength due to the shorter transverse relaxation times.

The ASL perfusion maps illustrated in **Fig. 90–1** were calculated from images acquired with a fast steady state free precession sequence (TrueFISP, with TR/TE = 4/2 msec and bandwidth = 651 Hz/pixel). Quantitative perfusion maps in units of mL·100 g^{-1}·min^{-1} can be calculated, as illustrated, if the tissue equilibrium magnetization is measured by means of a conventional proton density weighted image. The quantitative whole kidney perfusion maps displayed were acquired with a matrix of 192 × 192 and an in-plane resolution of 2 × 2 mm^2. The TrueFISP data acquisition offers similar SNR as compared with EPI, however, at notably lower sensitivity to magnetic field distortions. Shimming is advantageous, and a suitable scanner frequency has to be chosen providing TrueFISP images free of banding artifacts. The FAIR spin-labeling technique is typically applied in a single-slice mode, which is disadvantageous compared with conventional contrast-enhanced T1-weighted perfusion imaging. However, at 3 T the signal yield is sufficiently high to allow for acquisition of a single-slice perfusion map using FAIR within one

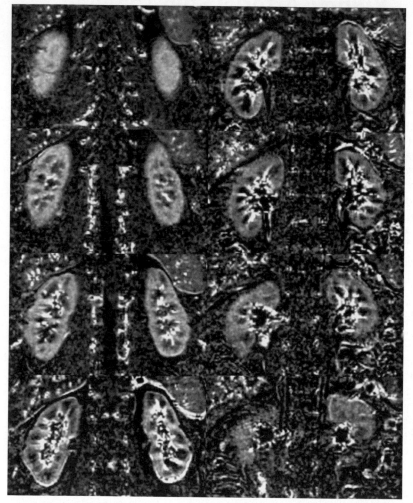

Figure 90–1

breath-hold. With sequential imaging of one slice during each breath-hold, the whole kidney can be mapped within less than 10 min. Altogether, the ASL technique is well suited for quantitative renal perfusion measurements, especially at high field strength (3 T).

91 Pelvis

Satoru Takahashi and Jurgen J. Fütterer

MR imaging is an established modality for the diagnosis of complex benign and malignant disorders of the pelvis. Whether for characterizing pelvic masses, identifying the extent of malignancies, preoperative planning, or determining post-treatment changes, MR has demonstrated itself to be an accurate and useful imaging technique. With 3 T, these clinical gains are only expected to be furthered.

Figures 91–1A to **91–1D** presents a comparison of images acquired at 1.5 T and 3 T in a 46-year-old woman with multiple leiomyomas. **(A)** At 1.5 T, axial T2-weighted images were acquired using FSE technique with TR/effective TE, 5516/116 msec; turbo factor, 17; flip angle, 150 degrees; and spatial resolution, $0.7 \times 0.7 \times 5$ mm $= 2.45$ mm^3 (voxel volume). **(B)** At 3 T, T2-weighted FSE images were obtained with TR/effective TE,

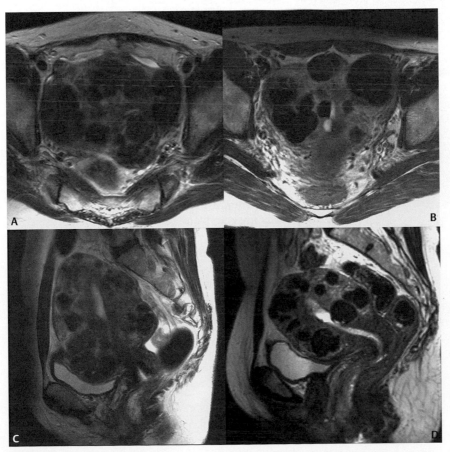

Figure 91–1

5060/101 msec; turbo factor, 15; flip angle, 120 degrees with hyperecho; and spatial resolution, $0.45 \times 0.45 \times 4$ mm $= 0.81$ mm^3 (voxel volume). Thanks to the high-resolution data acquisition, delineation of multiple intramural myomas is improved at 3 T when compared with 1.5 T, allowing for a more sophisticated evaluation of the leiomyoma, in terms of size, location, and characterization. This information has become important in the face of advances in uterine-conserving alternatives such as uterine artery embolization, hysteroscopic myomectomy, and hormone manipulation. To reduce SAR, a lower flip angle of 120 degrees was used at 3 T. Although hyperecho was applied to maintain T2 contrast, slight differences in tissue T2 contrast between 1.5 T and 3 T are seen. The (C) T2-weighted sagittal image at 1.5 T (TR/effective TE, 4640/109 msec) was acquired using an FSE sequence with high in-plane spatial resolution of 0.55×0.55 mm^2. Because a 5-mm slice thickness was used, the voxel volume was limited to 1.50 mm^3. To acquire (D), a 3D FSE sequence using a restore pulse and variable flip angle (SPACE) was applied at 3 T with an isotropic voxel of $0.98 \times 0.98 \times 0.98$ mm $= 0.93$ mm^3 (TR/effective TE $= 1100/115$ msec; turbo factor, 61; 2 echo trains per partition, iPAT of 3). Although the in-plane resolution of the 2D FSE scan at 1.5 T is higher than that of the 3D SPACE scan at 3 T, the voxel volume of the SPACE scan is smaller than that of the 2D FSE image due to the very thin section thickness of SPACE. Furthermore, multiplanar reformatted images in any imaging plane can be reconstructed using the

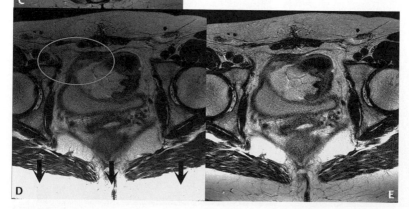

Figure 91–2

isotropic volume data set of the 3D SPACE scan. Although an extremely large turbo factor was applied in the SPACE sequence, use of a magnetization restore pulse and variable flip angle pulses along the echo train enable signal evolution largely identical to 2D FSE images.

Figures 91–2A to **91–2E** demonstrate the benefits and drawbacks of female pelvic imaging at 3 T in a 49-year-old woman with uterine cervical carcinoma. **Figure 91–2A** presents a 2D T2-weighted FSE image at 3 T (TR/effective TE, 5310/96 msec; turbo factor, 13; flip angle, 150 degrees; and spatial resolution, 0.45 × 0.45 × 3 mm = 0.61 mm³) successfully delineating the tumor in the uterine cervix (arrows), although contrast between the tumor and normal cervical stroma is poor. Shortened tissue T2 relaxation times and the lower flip angle used for reducing SAR can cause poor tissue T2 contrast at 3 T. **(B)** The 3D SPACE image (TR/effective TE = 1610/116 msec; turbo factor, 69; 2 echo trains per partition; iPAT of 3; and spatial resolution, 0.98 × 0.98 × 0.98 mm = 0.93 mm³) demonstrates lower spatial resolution and poorer contrast between the tumor and cervical stroma than 2D FSE images. **(C)** The transverse 2D T2-weighted FSE image with reduced spatial resolution (TR/effective TE, 3500/133 msec; turbo factor, 13; flip angle, 150 degrees; and spatial resolution, 0.78 × 0.78 × 3 mm = 1.55 mm³) demonstrates better contrast between the tumor (arrows) and normal cervical stroma.

Further optimization of scanning parameters for 3 T is needed to effectively image the pelvis. **(D)** The transverse 2D T2-weighted FSE image (TR/effective TE, 4500/96 msec; turbo factor, 13; flip angle, 150 degrees; and spatial resolution, 0.45 × 0.45 × 3 mm = 0.61 mm³) shows strong bright signal from dorsal subcutaneous fat tissue (arrows) and signal dropout (circle) anteriorly due to B_1 field inhomogeneity. **(E)** After application of a normalizing algorithm (bias field correction; BiFiC), homogeneity is improved.

92 Prostate: Introduction

Tom W.J. Scheenen

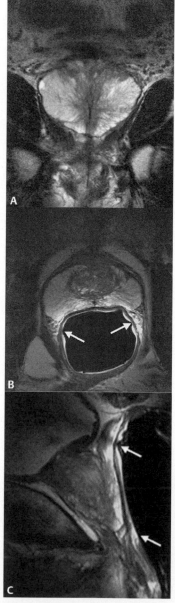

Figure 92–1

The basis for every MR imaging examination of prostate cancer patients is a detailed T2-weighted anatomical overview of the prostate in three dimensions. The use of an endorectal coil for signal reception at 3 T allows for an unprecedented spatial resolution within an acceptable measurement time. In **Fig. 92–1**, the voxel dimensions of the multislice FSE images are $0.26 \times 0.26 \times 2.5$ mm^3 [coronal (**A**) and axial (**B**)] and $0.35 \times 0.35 \times 4.0$ mm^3 [sagittal (**C**)]. In the scans presented, the TE was between 116 and 126 msec, whereas the acquisition time was respectively 3:02, 2:19, and 2:33 min:sec, depending on the number of slices and corresponding shortest TR. Correct positioning of the endorectal coil is crucial. With short localizers in sagittal and axial directions, both the depth and rotation of the endorectal balloon with the coil wiring inside (arrows in **Figs. 92–1B** and **92–1C**) can quickly be evaluated and, if necessary, adjusted. When imaging with an endorectal coil, the SNR changes dramatically with distance from the coil. Especially in images perpendicular to the coil wiring (**Figs. 92–1B** and **92–1C**) the SNR ranges from near zero to a maximum near or at the coil (arrows). To overcome a large signal drop in the images, a normalization filter is used in **Figs. 92–1B** and **92–1C**: signal intensities across the image become similar, but noise becomes more apparent at larger distances from the coil.

The use of the endorectal coil in MR of the prostate is a point of debate: the coil causes discomfort for the patient, requires additional MR scanner time for insertion and evaluation of the correct position, and is expensive (the coil itself and the additional MR time). An alternative at 3 T is the use of combined multiple array elements from the spine and body array coils for signal reception. In **Fig. 92–2**, T2-weighted FSE images of the same patient as in **Fig. 92–1** at the same position are shown. Matrix size and FOV need to be adopted to avoid wraparound: the resulting voxel dimensions are $0.5 \times 0.5 \times 4.0$ mm^3 for all images. With two averages, the acquisition time ranges from 3:33 to 3:54 min:sec and the echo time is 127 msec for all directions [coronal **(A)**, axial **(B)**, and sagittal **(C)**]. If one is interested in more than just the prostate, the external array coils are the obvious choice for signal reception. If it is really only the prostate one is interested in, one can consider the additional effort of using the endorectal coil, offering the highest SNR inside the prostate possible at 3 T.

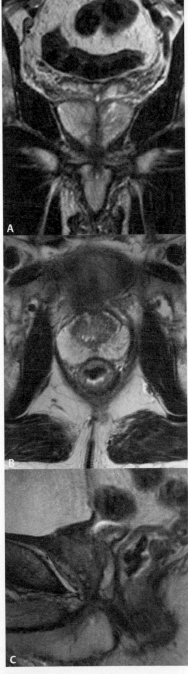

Figure 92–2

93 Prostate: Anatomy

Tom W.J. Scheenen

For accurate local staging of prostate cancer, it is important to have the best anatomical detail available. In **Fig. 93–1,** axial T2-weighted FSE images of a prostate from apex to base at 3 T are shown with a spatial resolution of 0.26 × 0.26 × 2.5 mm³, acquired in 3:02 min:sec at TE 116 msec (same patient as in Case 92). The prostate capsule is clearly delineated at the edge of the peripheral zone that encompasses the central gland (outlined in **Fig. 93–1H**). On T2-weighted MR imaging, prostate cancer often occurs as a low signal intensity lesion. Because diseases other than cancer can enlarge especially the central gland of the prostates of older men, a lesion on T2-weighted MR imaging alone is not a very specific marker for prostate cancer. If, however, a lesion is detected in combination with disruption or bulging of the prostate capsule or invasion of the seminal vesicles, the tissue is suspect for T3 prostate cancer, involving different treatment strategies than locally confined disease stage T2. In **Fig. 93–2,** the benefit of increased field strength in staging the disease is illustrated. A 64-year-old patient with biopsy-proven prostate cancer underwent T2-weighted FSE MR imaging at both 1.5 and 3 T. At 1.5 T (**Figs. 93–2A and 93–2D),** the voxel size was 0.35 × 0.35 × 4.0 mm³ with a TE of 119 msec. At 3 T, an equal voxel size and TE was used in **Figs. 93–2B** and **93–2E,** and a voxel size of 0.18 × 0.18 × 2.5 mm³ with a

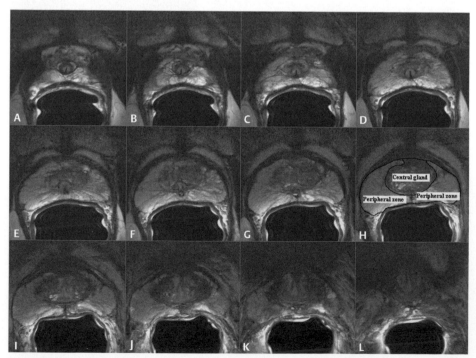

Figure 93–1

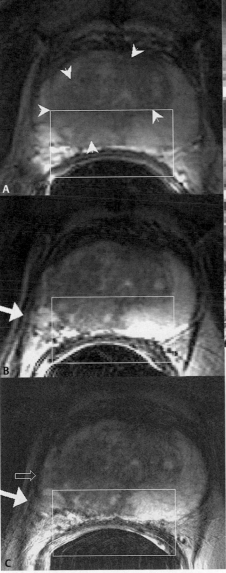

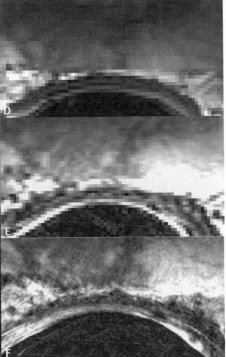

Figure 93–2

TE of 162 msec was used for **Figs. 93–2C** and **93–2F**, after adoption of matrix size, number of slices, and TR, making full use of the increased SNR. At 3 T, hyperechoes were also used to reduce SAR. In all prostate images, a lesion is visible in the central gland and right peripheral zone (arrowheads in **Fig. 93–2A**). Bulging of the capsule by a hyperintense structure is visible in the right peripheral zone (solid white arrow in **Figs. 93–2B** and **93–2C**), and in the high-resolution image, lack of definition of the prostate capsule next to the lesion can be discerned (open arrow in **Fig. 93–2C**), indicating extracapsular extension of the tumor. Figures **93–2D** to **93–2F** are a magnification of the boxes in **Figs. 93–2A** to **93–2C**, respectively. When zooming in on images for precise evaluation of prostate delineation, one can best appreciate the increase in anatomical detail (**Fig. 93–2F** compared with **Figs. 93–2D** and **93–2E**) when making full use of the available SNR with an endorectal coil at 3 T.

94 Prostate: Contrast-Enhanced Imaging

Tom W.J. Scheenen

Contrast-enhanced imaging with low-molecular-weight agents, specifically the gadolinium chelates, relies on the T1-shortening properties of the contrast agent molecules, perfusion of the tissue under investigation, and the local ability of the contrast agent molecules to extravasate out of the blood vessels into the extracellular space. Tumor tissue often has increased perfusion over healthy tissue, as newly formed blood vessels try to supply the growing tumor with oxygen and nutrients. Moreover, these new blood vessels, lacking refined structure, can be disrupted and leaky. Therefore, tumor tissue can be visualized with T1-weighted MR imaging after contrast agent administration. Because T2-weighted imaging of anatomy alone (Case 93) may not be very specific for the detection and localization of prostate cancer, T1-weighted MR imaging acts as an independent additional marker. In **Fig. 94–1,** the anatomy of the prostate of a 65-year-old patient (PSA level 25 μg/L) with biopsy-proven prostate cancer (total Gleason grade 5) is visualized from apex to base with multislice T2-weighted FSE MR imaging at 3 T; voxel size was $0.26 \times 0.26 \times 2.5$ mm^3 with a TE of 153 msec, acquisition time 3 min. In the images of the bottom row, the bladder is visible, and the circular structures just above the coil in the final image are the seminal vesicles. A large lesion is visible in the base on the right side of the prostate, extending into the seminal vesicles (arrows in **Fig. 94–1**). The central gland of the prostate consists of heterogeneous tissue with large differences in intensity. After an intravenous bolus

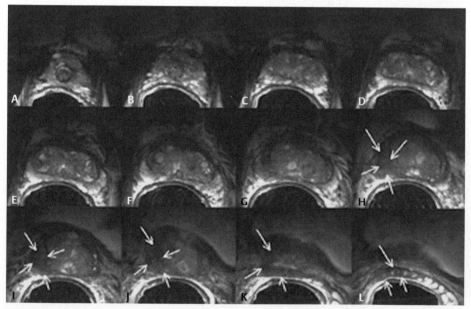

Figure 94–1

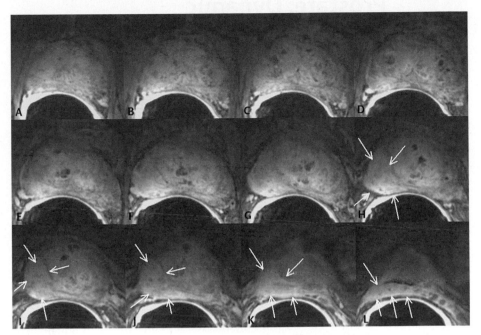

Figure 94–2

injection of paramagnetic gadolinium chelate, the lesion in the base of the prostate in **Fig. 94–1** enhances on T1-weighted imaging. In **Fig. 94–2**, 12 images from a 3D series of 32 images are shown with the enhancing lesion indicated with arrows. A 3D T1-weighted GRE sequence was used with TR 8.6 msec and flip angle 15 degrees; the voxel size was $0.5 \times 0.5 \times 1.5$ mm^3 and TE 4 msec. With the TR and flip angle used, intracellular water or, generally, water that is not in contact with the contrast agent will be saturated and therefore hypointense. Water that is in contact with the contrast agent will not, or will only partially be, saturated and become hyperintense, enhancing the tissue in which the highest concentrations of contrast agent occur. Especially for inexperienced readers, the addition of contrast-enhanced imaging will add confidence to assigning tumor tissue to lesions on T2-weighted MR imaging that extend beyond the prostate capsule or into the seminal vesicles. As in Case 93, the combination of an endorectal coil and a field strength of 3 T provides the best anatomical detail possible at this moment in prostate MR imaging. An additional advantage of using an endorectal coil in 3D imaging is the fact that the FOV can be made much smaller and dedicated to the prostate, as no signal is measured from tissue at large distances from the balloon, so no wraparound will occur.

95 Prostate: Dynamic Contrast-Enhanced Imaging

Tom W.J. Scheenen

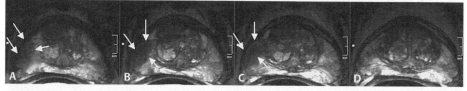

Figure 95–1

Dynamic contrast-enhanced MR imaging (DCE MRI) is a method to sample the dynamic aspects of contrast agent administration. Apart from differences in contrast enhancement between healthy and tumor tissue on a time scale of several min, as discussed in Case 94, DCE MRI zooms in on the first pass of the contrast agent through the tissue. **Figs. 95–1** and **95–2,** the anatomical basis of an MR study (see Case 93) of a 58-year-old patient with prostate cancer, reveal a lesion in the right peripheral zone of the prostate in both axial (**Fig. 95–1**) and coronal (**Fig. 95–2**) planes, indicated with the arrows. After an intravenous bolus injection of paramagnetic gadolinium chelate (at a dose of 0.1 mmol/kg) using a power injector with an injection rate of 2.5 mL/sec followed by 15-mL saline flush, the contrast agent entering the tissue is visualized for 2 min with a fast 3D T1-weighted GRE sequence with a TE of 1.6 msec, TR 3.8 msec, and flip angle 10 degrees. With partial Fourier encoding in two phase-encoding dimensions, a temporal resolution of 1 sec for a 3D volume could be reached (voxel size $1.1 \times 2.2 \times 4.0$ mm^3). For every individual voxel of the 3D volume, a signal intensity versus time curve can be constructed and analyzed with curve fitting or pharmacokinetic modeling. In **Fig. 95–3,** the relative contrast agent concentration in time of a voxel in healthy and in tumor tissue are plotted on the same scale. Generally, in tumor tissue the contrast agent concentration rapidly reaches a maximum value that is larger than maximum values in healthy tissues and decreases again within the 2-min time window. After modeling these curves, pharmacokinetic maps can be overlaid on the T2-weighted images, as is done in **Fig. 95–4** (see **Color Plate 95–4**) (courtesy of Stijn W. Heijmink, M.D.). From top to bottom, the following maps are shown: washout (**A**) characterizes the negative slope of the signal intensity curve after the initial maximum enhancement. Kep (**B**) is the rate constant of

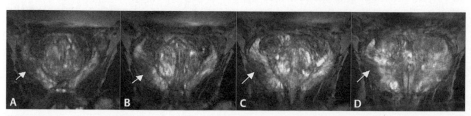

Figure 95–2

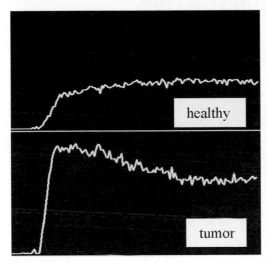

Figure 95–3

exchange of contrast agent between blood plasma on the one hand and extracellular/extravascular space V **(C)** on the other. Ktrans [axial **(D)** and coronal **(E)**] is the volume transfer constant of contrast agent exchange. All these parameters have increased values within the lesion in **Figs. 95–1** and **95–2**. However, apart from the tumor focus, other small areas also enhance: the exact sensitivities and specificities of the different parameters are still under investigation. Generally, the sensitivity of DCE-MRI is quite high, but it may lack specificity.

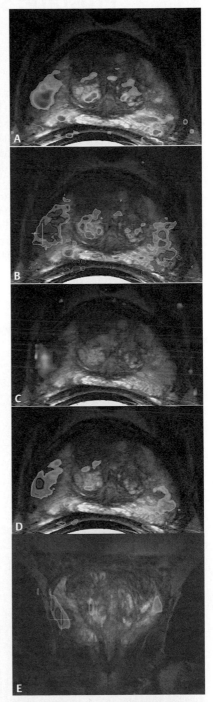

Figure 95–4 (See Color Plate 95–4.)

96 Prostate: Spectroscopy

Tom W.J. Scheenen

Spectroscopic imaging (SI) of the prostate gives insight into the presence of certain metabolites in the different tissues. With a ^{1}H-spectroscopic imaging experiment, a spectrum is acquired from every voxel of a user-defined 3D volume of interest (VOI) around the prostate. In **Fig. 96–1A,** one slab of the SI matrix is overlaid on a 3 T axial T2-weighted image of a 70-year-old patient with prostate cancer in the left central gland. The white box around the prostate is the VOI; the four white slabs are saturation slabs to suppress signals from these regions, as the prostate is embedded in lipid tissue that gives rise to intense unwanted signals. From two voxels inside the VOI, a typical healthy spectrum (right peripheral zone) is shown in **Fig. 96–1C,** and a typical spectrum from tumor tissue (left central gland) is shown in **Fig. 96–1D.** Four metabolite signals are present and identified at fixed positions in the spectra: the ratio of choline over citrate is used as a marker for tumor tissue. In **Fig. 96–1B,** the relevant parts of the spectra of every voxel

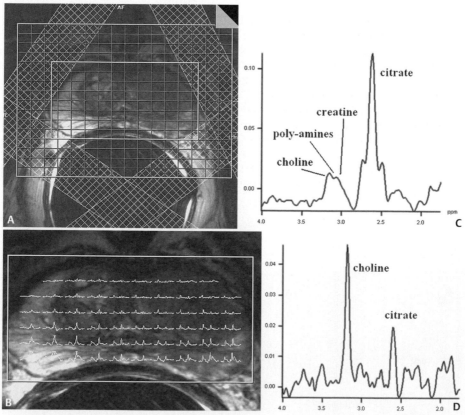

Figure 96–1

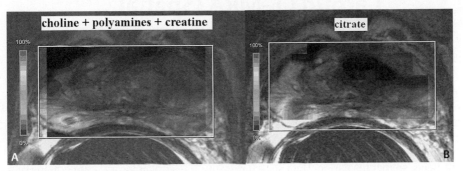

Figure 96–2 (See Color Plate 96–2.)

are plotted onto the T2-weighted image. Because an endorectal coil has been used, the metabolite signal intensities decrease with distance from the coil.

Metabolite ratios (SNR permitted), however, do not depend on this distance. In **Fig. 96–2** (see **Color Plate 96–2**), the total signal intensity of combined choline, creatine, and polyamines **(A)** and the total citrate signal **(B)** are presented in a color overlay on the T2-weighted image. The loss of signal intensity with increasing distance from the coil is evident. The overlaid color maps are strongly interpolated: the true size of a voxel from the SI experiment can best be approximated by a sphere with radius 5 mm and corresponding volume 0.5 cm^3 (other SI parameters: TE/TR 145/750 msec, acquisition time 8.5 min with so-called weighted averaging). As the separation of the different resonances in the spectra is field strength dependent, it is now possible at 3 T to construct interpolated color maps of the ratio of solely choline over citrate, which could be an even more specific marker for tumor tissue. For the same patient as in **Figs. 96–1** and **96–2,** these ratio maps are constructed in **Fig. 96–3** (see **Color Plate 96–3**) in an axial **(A)** and coronal **(B)** plane, overlaid on the T2-weighted images. All over the left central gland, the choline-to-citrate ratio is elevated compared with the remainder of the prostate. The sensitivity and specificity for detecting prostate cancer using an absolute threshold value of the ratio needs to be evaluated in large patient populations.

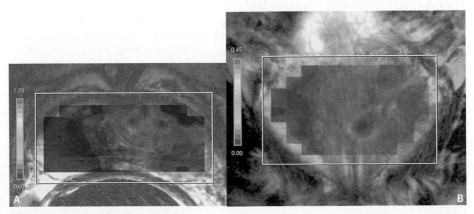

Figure 96–3 (See Color Plate 96–3.)

97 Carotid CE-MRA (Spatial Resolution)

Benjamin Hyman and Val M. Runge

Contrast-enhanced MRA (CE-MRA) has become the modality of choice for evaluation of the head and neck arteries during the past decade. Clear advantages include the noninvasive nature of the procedure, the lack of ionizing radiation, the large provided FOV, and the decreased (negligible) risk of ischemic injury (versus catheter angiography). There are some limitations to the exam when performed at 1.5 T, with likely the most important being spatial resolution. High spatial resolution is critical for accurate grading of a stenosis, with resultant impact on therapeutic decision-making based on the North American Symptomatic Carotid Endarterectomy Trial (NASCET) criteria. Improved spatial resolution could come from decreasing the FOV, but that would limit the visualization of tandem stenoses that might exist along the course of the vessels, from the aortic arch to the intracranial circulation. Other gains in resolution from increased time of acquisition are met with increased likelihood of patient movement or venous contamination limiting the study. With advances in parallel imaging, both spatial and temporal resolution improvements could be achieved, but not without a critical SNR penalty at 1.5 T. With the advent of 3 T, due to the high available SNR, the performance of carotid CE-MRA can be substantially improved. Clear differences are seen due to voxel size reduction and improved spatial resolution without prolonged scan times. Alternatively, scan times can be reduced by ~50% with little loss in image resolution. **Figures 97–1A** to **97–1C** demonstrate, with coronal, sagittal, and axial MIPs from a 3 T CE-MRA exam using a parallel imaging (IPAT) factor of 4, how high spatial resolution allows for significant improvements in accuracy and grading of stenoses. Seen on this study of an 87-year-old man with atherosclerosis is a severe stenosis (arrow) at the origin of the left internal carotid artery, well depicted due to the high spatial resolution. Overestimation of stenosis has been an issue with larger voxel size and partial volume effects at 1.5 T.

Figures 97–2A and **97–2B** present sagittal MIP images from a CE-MRA exam at 3 T with IPAT factors of 2 and 4, respectively, in the same subject.

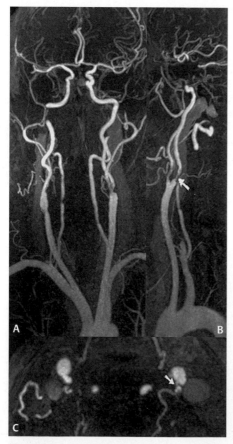

Figure 97–1

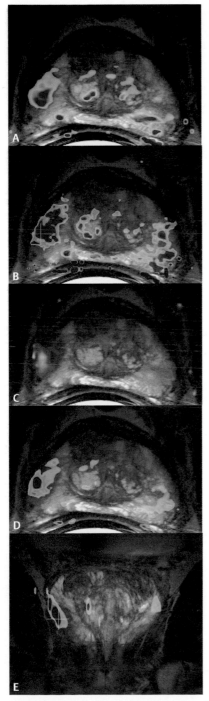

Color Plate 95–4 (See Figure 95–4, page 217.)

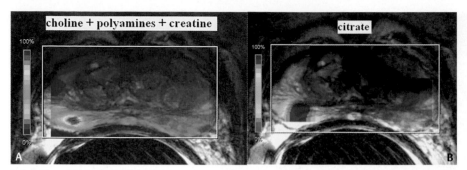

Color Plate 96–2 (See Figure 96–2, page 219.)

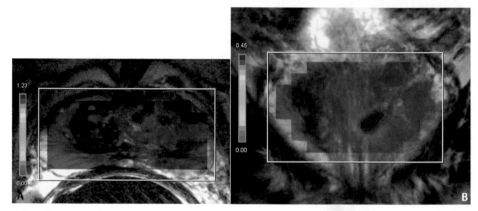

Color Plate 96–3 (See Figure 96–3, page 219.)

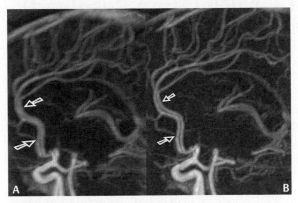

Figure 97–2

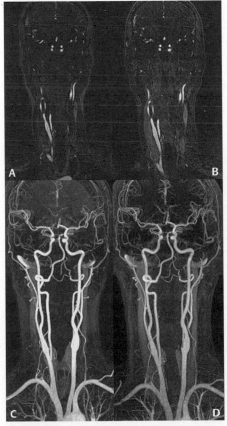

Figure 97–3

Demonstrated in this figure is the difference that improved spatial resolution provides, in this instance the ability to clearly separate the two closely opposed anterior cerebral arteries (arrows). At 1.5 T, at most an acceleration factor of 2 can be applied, due to lower SNR, limiting available spatial resolution relative to 3 T.

When looking at the source data alone from 3 T (**Figs. 97–3A** and **97–3B**), there is substantially lower SNR when an IPAT of 4 (**B**) is used versus an IPAT of 2 (**A**). However, as seen in **Figs. 97–3C** and **97–3D**, with the corresponding MIP reconstructions, the decrease in SNR does not substantially degrade depiction of the arterial vessels.

Figures 97-1, 97-2, and 97-3 from Nael K, Ruehm SG, Michaely HJ, Pope W, Laub G, Finn JP, et al. High spatial-resolution CE-MRA of the carotid circulation with parallel imaging: comparison of image quality between 2 different acceleration factors at 3.0 tesla. Invest Radiol 2006;41: 391–399. Reprinted by permission.

98   Carotid CE-MRA (Time-Resolved)

Benjamin Hyman and Val M. Runge

Time-resolved CE-MRA suffers from limitations in temporal and spatial resolution due to the very nature of the acquisition, which requires following the contrast bolus as it passes through the arterial and venous circulation. By combining the faster acquisition times and larger FOV made possible by parallel imaging with the improved SNR attributes of 3 T, the quality of dynamic carotid studies has improved substantially. Recent studies have demonstrated temporal resolutions as high as 1.5 sec. With rapid arteriovenous transits, high temporal resolution is important for disease diagnosis in many instances, for example subclavian steal. An added benefit from parallel imaging with 3 T is the ability to demonstrate good temporal and spatial resolution without limiting the FOV, with visualization of both aortic and intracranial vessels possible in a single exam.

Figure 98–1 demonstrates the combination of dynamic information with high spatial resolution that can be attained using 3 T with aggressive parallel imaging. Illustrated is a dynamic MIP series from a time-resolved 3 T CE-MRA showing a high-grade stenosis at the origin of the brachiocephalic artery with reversal of flow through the right vertebral artery and resultant right subclavian steal.

Figure 98–2 presents a dynamic MIP study in the coronal plane, with each image 1.8 sec in duration, that reveals a large left middle cerebral artery feeding an

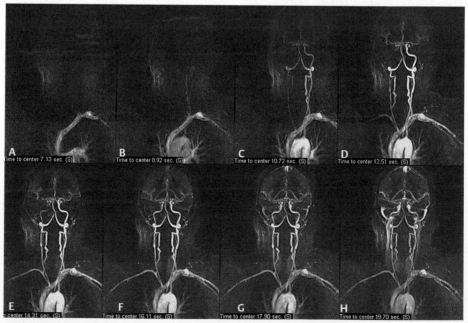

Figure 98–1

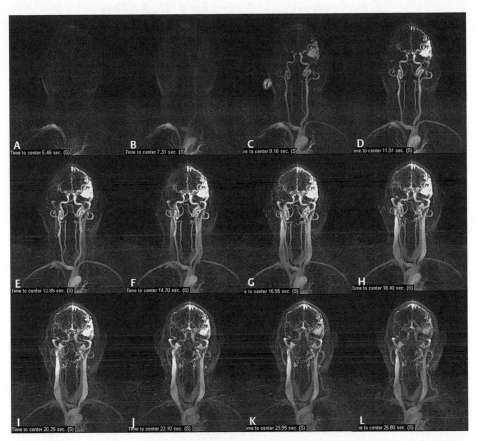

Figure 98–2

arteriovenous malformation in the left temporal lobe. Associated superficial venous drainage can also be seen. Well illustrated is the large FOV, with the possibility of visualization of pathology from the level of the aortic arch to and including the intracranial vessels.

In summary, 3 T is effective in supporting fast acquisition protocols by use of the available high SNR, making possible improved spatial and temporal resolution. This in turn provides a tremendously helpful tool in fast dynamic imaging of the carotids and other smaller vessels with fast flow.

Figures 98–1 and 98–2 from Nael K, Michaely HJ, Villablanca P, Salamon N, Laub G, Finn JP. Time-resolved contrast enhanced magnetic resonance angiography of the head and neck at 3.0 tesla: initial results. Invest Radiol 2006;41:116–124. Reprinted by permission.

99 Abdominal Aortic CE-MRA (Resolution)

Henrik J. Michaely

Table 99–1   Typical MRA Parameters

	1.5 T MRA	3 T MRA	Change
TR/TE (ms)	3.77/1.39	3.14/1.1	↓ by 17/21%
Flip angle (degrees)	25	23	↔
Bandwidth (Hz/pixel)	350	510	↑ by 45%
Matrix	512 × 410	512 × 410	↔
FOV (mm²)	400 × 348	400 × 324	↔
Phase oversampling (%)	0	8	
Voxel size (mm³)	0.8	0.65	↓ by 19%
Spatial resolution (mm³)	1 × 0.8 × 1	0.9 × 0.8 × 0.9	
Scan time (s)	27	18	↓ by 34%
Partitions/3D volume	80	96	↑ by 8%
Parallel imaging	GRAPPA 2	GRAPPA 3	

Due to the doubling of SNR, abdominal MRA at 3 T holds promise for fast imaging with high spatial resolution. Compared with 1.5 T, the readout bandwidth can be increased at 3 T to further minimize the TR, however a further decrease in TR is restricted by safety restraints (peripheral nerve stimulation and SAR). The application of parallel imaging (GRAPPA, factor of three, left to right) makes possible an unprecedented increase in spatial resolution (matrix and slice thickness). The administration of high-relaxivity contrast agents (Gd-BOPTA, Bracco) or 1.0-molar contrast agents (Gadobutrol, Schering) additionally compensates for the SNR drop associated with higher spatial resolution and higher parallel imaging factors. Compared with a state-of-the-art protocol for abdominal MRA at 1.5 T, 3 T MRA achieves higher spatial resolution and larger volume coverage in a drastically decreased scan time (**Table 99–1**). Due to the shorter scan times, faster injection of the contrast agent is however warranted.

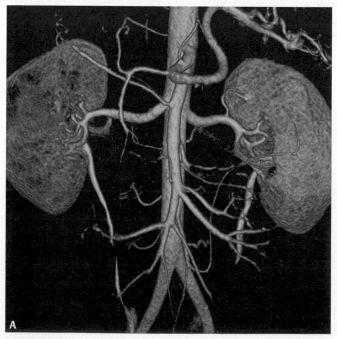

Figure 99–1

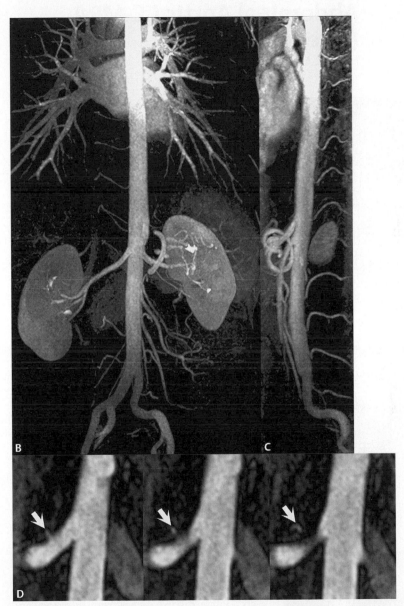

Figure 99–1 *(Continued)*

Imaging with this approach leads to multidetector CT-like image quality (**Fig. 99–1A**) over the entire FOV of 50 cm (**Fig. 99–1B**). The high level of depicted details can be appreciated in **Fig. 99–1C,** where all the lumbar arteries are well visualized. The high spatial resolution and short scan time, which minimizes motion artifact, permit the display of even the smallest vascular structures, such as the tiny vessel branch demonstrated (**Fig. 99–1D,** arrows).

Abdominal Aortic CE-MRA (Aneurysm)

Henrik J. Michaely

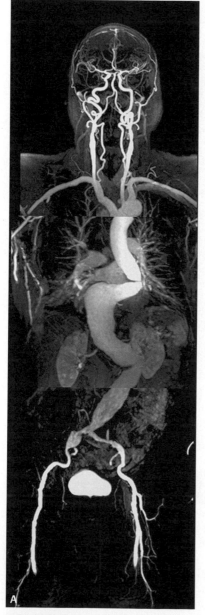

Figure 100–1

In the past decade, MRA has evolved into a standard tool for evaluation of abdominal atherosclerotic vessel disease, including renal artery stenosis, aortic aneurysms, and stenoses of the mesenterial arteries. Other major sites of atherosclerosis are the carotid arteries and the peripheral arteries. In contrast with CTA, severe calcifications do not hamper the assessment of the vessel lumen significantly. Only in cases of very pronounced calcifications may a signal void occur in MRA. However, this rarely interferes with image quality and image interpretation. The patient shown in the images (**Figs. 100–1A** to **100–1C**) suffers from severe hypertension and was suspected to have both a carotid artery stenosis and an aortic aneurysm. A protocol with two injections of contrast agent was chosen to image the carotid arteries with the first bolus and the abdomen and pelvis with the second bolus. The large FOV that current 3 T scanners offer allows for overlapping 3D volumes from which **Fig. 100–1A** is composed. No carotid artery stenosis was found. However, an extremely elongated and kinked aorta with partial thrombosis (**Fig. 100–1B**, arrows) and aneurysmal changes is well delineated. In addition, a moderate-grade stenosis of the celiac axis was found (**Fig. 100–1C**). Although **Fig. 100–1A** suggests the existence of right-sided renal artery stenosis, no renal artery stenosis was noted on oblique reformats parallel to the vessel axis.

Aneurysmal changes as shown in this example can pose technical problems for MR technologists. Flow disturbances from kinking and aneurysms may render correct bolus timing impossible. In these cases, time-resolved MRA studies can be applied. At 3 T, a high temporal resolution of 1.6 sec per 3D volume can be achieved with dedicated sequences using view-sharing and parallel imaging. In contrast with 1.5 T, the spatial resolution of these dynamic scans can be kept at a high level of 1.5 × 1.5 × 3.0 mm³.

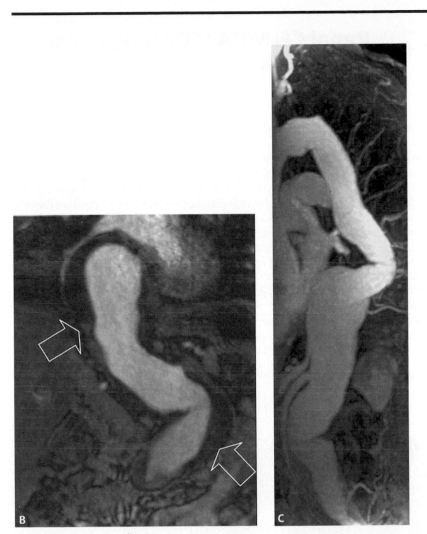

Figure 100–1 *(Continued)*

Dynamic studies are of particular value in patients with aortic dissections to demonstrate the blood flow dynamics, determine the reentry site, and assess organ perfusion. But they are also of interest in patients suffering from congenital vascular malformations such as major aortopulmonary collateral artery (MAPCA), which often are easily visible on time-resolved studies because of their characteristic irregular nature. In high-resolution static MRA, these irregular vessels may be hidden by overlying normal vessels.

101 Renal CE-MRA (Fibromuscular Dysplasia)

Henrik J. Michaely

Fibromuscular dysplasia (FMD) is a rare cause of renal artery stenosis, accounting for less than 10% of cases. It occurs primarily in young women. The most common FMD type, medial fibroplasia, is characterized by the classical "string of beads" appearance of the affected vessel, with the "beads" usually larger than the adjacent normal vessel caliber. Other types of FMD exhibit beads that are smaller than the normal vessel caliber. Pathologic vessel wall changes can be focal, include one entire renal artery, or include both (38%) renal arteries. Due to the vessel wall weakness in FMD, FMD accounts for 38% of all renal artery aneurysms and is responsible for a major part of renal artery dissections. FMD affects mainly the middle and distal third of the renal arteries whereas the proximal part is involved in only 30% of cases. This is one reason why FMD is still a challenge for 3D contrast-enhanced MRA, as the distal part of the renal artery shows considerable motion from random diaphragmatic motion, independent of breath holding. Another reason is that the dysplastic vessel sections can be very subtle and focal. Conventional angiography as the current gold standard has an in-plane resolution of up to 300 μm, whereas even high-resolution CE-MRA at 1.5 T hardly surpasses 1000 μm.

The high SNR at 3 T now allows fast imaging with high spatial resolution. This approach largely eliminates motion-related artifacts and provides high spatial resolution even for the distal parts of the renal arteries. For the patient shown in **Fig. 101–1A.** (with the close-up, **Fig. 101–1B**), a fast 3D-FLASH sequence with a spatial resolution of

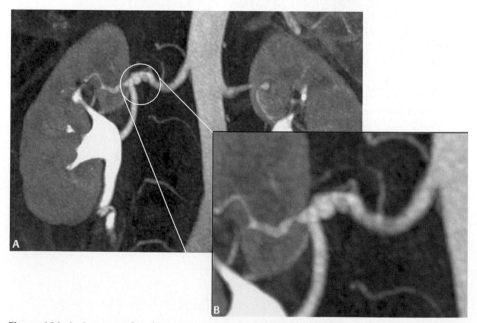

Figure 101–1 Courtesy of Paul Finn, University of California, Los Angeles.

0.9 × 0.8 × 0.9 mm³ and 16-sec acquisition time was used. The typical string of beads becomes clearly visible in the distal third of the main renal artery. This example demonstrates that the technical capabilities at 3 T will allow better visualization of the distal renal arteries. In this role, 3 T MRA will perform substantially better than currently used techniques at 1.5 T. A slightly different approach was chosen in the patient shown in **Figs. 101–1C** and **101–1D** who also suffered from FMD but exhibited multiple unilateral renal artery aneurysms instead of the typical string of beads. In this patient, a contrast-enhanced MRA with a non-isotropic spatial resolution of 0.9 × 0.6 × 1.4 mm³ was chosen to cover a larger slab with high in-plane resolution. Even though this approach provides higher SNR due to the thicker slab, it may be unfavorable when reformats are used, as the images will demonstrate blurring in the direction of the lowest resolution.

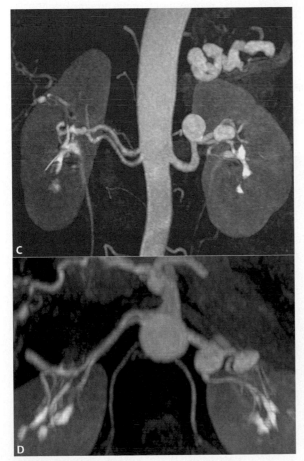

Figure 101–1 *(Continued)*

Peripheral CE-MRA (Part 1)

Harald Kramer

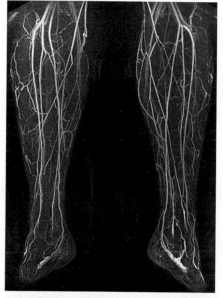

Figure 102–1

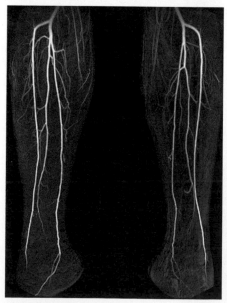

Figure 102–2

Magnetic resonance angiography (MRA) has become the new gold standard for evaluation of the vasculature of the lower extremities, although it still suffers from some restrictions in terms of image quality. To acquire a complete angiogram of the lower body, the abdominal aorta must be imaged from the diaphragm caudally to include the arteries of the calves and feet. Up to now, this has only been possible in three to four consecutive steps, in which the problem of venous enhancement arises in the most distal station **(Fig. 102–1)**. To avoid this, the acquisition time of the more proximal stations has to be kept at a minimum, resulting in limited spatial resolution. Parallel acquisition techniques (PAT) help to reduce acquisition time while maintaining spatial resolution, at the cost of SNR. At 3 T, this reduction in SNR is less of a problem than at 1.5 T, given the increased SNR at the higher field. The improvement in SNR with field strength can be used in different ways when performing MRA of the peripheral arteries. Certainly, acquisition time can be reduced, but a scan duration of ~20 sec is feasible, even in elderly patients for breath-hold acquisitions. On the other hand, spatial resolution can be further increased in the more proximal MRA stations for good depiction of the renal and iliac arteries. In the most distal MRA station, when breath-hold times do not matter anymore, the higher available SNR can be used solely to increase spatial resolution. Thus it is not only possible to image the three main arteries of the calf but also the small side branches **(Fig. 102–2)**. For therapy planning, it is important to image the small pedal arteries as a target for distal anastomosis in peripheral arterial occlusive disease (PAOD). To further increase spatial

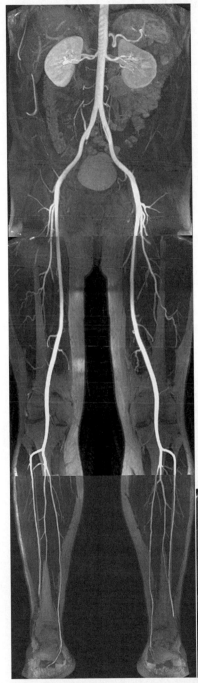

resolution and reduce acquisition time, dedicated array coils should be used.

When using modern multichannel MR systems in combination with multielement coils, PAT acceleration factors of up to four are possible. This allows for submillimeter spatial resolution within a 20-sec acquisition time. For the abdominal station, TR of 3.31, TE of 1.21, flip angle of 30 degrees, 448 matrix size, 88 slices/slab, and 400 Hz/pixel bandwidth result in a spatial resolution of $1.4 \times 1.1 \times 1.2$ mm^3 in an acquisition time of 18 sec with a PAT acceleration factor of three. For the thigh station, these parameters change to TR 3.51 and TE 1.33. Flip angle and number of slices/slab remain unchanged, matrix size is increased to 512, bandwidth to 410 Hz/pixel, providing a spatial resolution of 1 mm^3 isotropic within an acquisition time of 15 sec using a PAT acceleration factor of four. For MRA of the calves, TR is 3.98, TE is 1.47, and the matrix size is further increased to 576 with 104 slices/slab and a bandwidth of 330 Hz/pixel. Here a spatial resolution of 0.9 mm^3 isotropic within a scan time of 23 sec can be reached (**Fig. 102–3**).

When using blood pool contrast agents, acquisition time is less important because there is no need for arterial timing. Here, spatial resolution can be increased to $0.6 \times 0.6 \times 0.6$ mm^3 for a 2:01 min:sec acquisition time (**Fig. 102–4**).

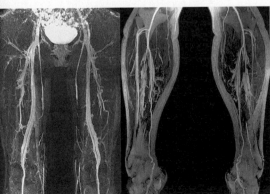

Figure 102–3

Figure 102–4

103   Peripheral CE-MRA (Part 2)
Harald Kramer

Up to now, noninvasive methods for imaging the arterial vasculature including specifically CTA and MRA have suffered from reduced temporal resolution compared with digital subtraction angiography (DSA). Multiphasic MRA offered dynamic information that was not sufficient for a diagnostic exam. To obtain the information needed concerning flow characteristics in patients with stenotic lesions or occlusions, a temporal resolution of less than 4 sec is needed. This information can have a tremendous impact on treatment planning because with this technique it can be clarified how blood (contrast agent) reaches the more distal vessels. This is of great importance in interventional planning (e.g., before bypass surgery or shunting in patients undergoing hemodialysis). When increasing the temporal resolution of an MRA exam, spatial resolution and SNR naturally decreases. High field strength and dedicated angiography coils help to maintain image quality, at the level achieved with standard MRA procedures at 1.5 T, or even to increase it while enhancing temporal resolution. When applying a PAT acceleration factor of three at 3 T and using a dedicated 32-element angiography coil, a temporal resolution of 3.5 sec/slab is feasible **(Fig. 103–1)**. When applying a PAT factor of four, a temporal resolution of 2.9 sec/slab is possible **(Fig. 103–2)**. Spatial resolution in these exams is 1.4 × 1.4 × 1.5 mm³. The remaining parameters are TR 2.27 and TE 0.81, FOV 360 mm, matrix

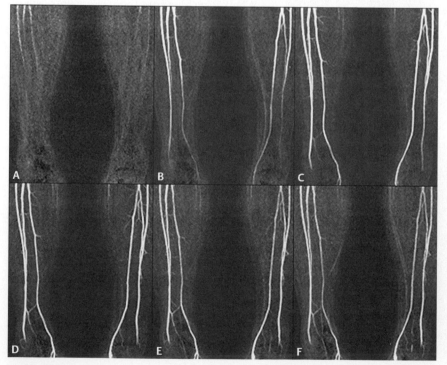

Figure 103–1

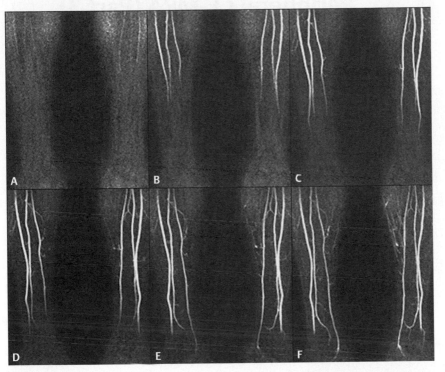

Figure 103–2

of 256^2, flip angle 16 degrees, 48 slices/slab, and bandwidth of 890 Hz/pixel. The combination of PAT and high temporal resolution is possible with dedicated angiography sequences that employ view sharing like in TREAT (time-resolved echo-shared angiography technique). At 3 T, high SNR can be preserved in time-resolved images despite the relatively high spatial resolution. **Figure 103–3** shows a comparison of a static high-resolution first-pass MRA **(A)** with a time-resolved MRA **(B)** in the same patient.

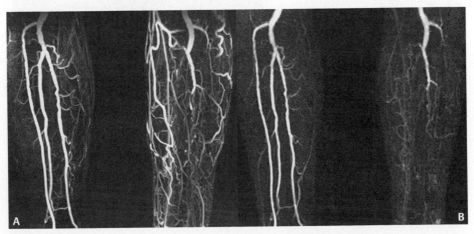

Figure 103–3

Peripheral CE-MRA (Part 3)

Harald Kramer

The images presented in this case were acquired from a patient suffering from long-standing diabetes mellitus and PAOD Fontaine/Rutherford grade 3, with a painless walking distance of 50 m. A Y-prosthesis of the aortic bifurcation was implanted 3 years prior to the current exam. Imaging was performed to clarify if there is the possibility of surgical treatment, including specifically bypass surgery. In this case, it is important to assess if there are vessel occlusions with well-perfused arteries more distal to the occlusion or if the vessels are just fading away without distal reconstitution. It is also important to see if there is quick shunting to draining veins caused by chronic inflammatory disease. The MRA protocol should be adapted to these questions. When using a blood pool contrast agent, the complete lower body should be imaged in the first pass to display the abdominal aorta, the Y-prosthesis, and the peripheral vasculature of the legs **(Fig. 104–1)**. In the steady state, images of the regions of interest (e.g., vessel segments with pathologic changes) should be acquired

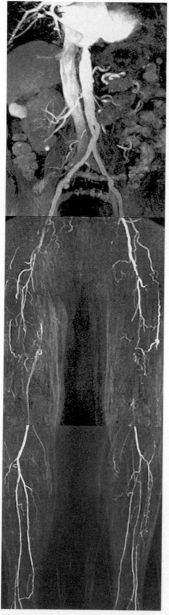

Figure 104–1

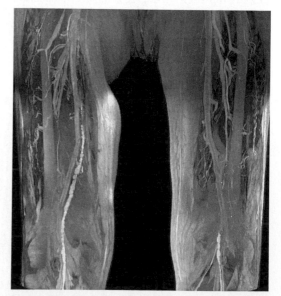

Figure 104–2

(**Fig. 104–2**). In vessel segments, which are suited for a distal anastomosis of a bypass graft, spatial resolution should be increased as much as possible, given the limitations of SNR. While performing first-pass MRA, spatial resolution of the abdominal aorta of less than $1.5 \times 1.5 \times 1.5$ mm^3 is sufficient. In the more distal stations, spatial resolution should be increased to be less than 1.2 mm^3. Steady-state MRA of target vessel segments for treatment should provide submillimeter isotropic resolution. In the case presented, the spatial resolution is $1.4 \times 1.1 \times 1.5$ mm^3 in the abdominal first-pass MRA and $1 \times 1 \times 1$ mm^3 and $0.9 \times 0.9 \times 0.9$ mm^3, respectively, in the first-pass MRA of the thigh and calf stations. In every station, the acquisition time was less than 20 sec. Spatial resolution of the steady-state MRA of the thigh is $0.8 \times 0.8 \times 0.8$ mm^3 with an acquisition time of 25 sec. In comparison with DSA (**Fig. 104–3**), MRA (**Fig. 104–4**) can better display small distal arteries sufficient for anastomosis. DSA and MRA show an occlusion of the superficial femoral artery on both sides (**Fig. 104–4A**). In the iliac vessels, a stenosis at the anastomosis can be detected on the left side; the right-sided anastomosis shows a small aneurysm (**Fig. 104–4B**).

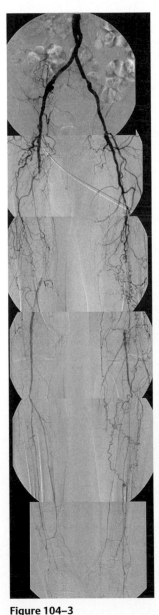

Figure 104–3

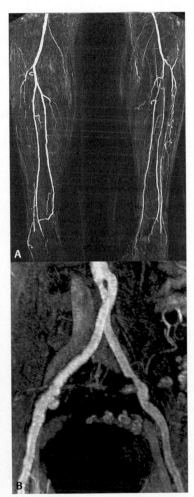

Figure 104–4

Index

Page numbers followed by an italic *f* or *t* indicate the entry on that page is in a figure or table.